Medical Device Design and Regulation

Also available from ASQ Quality Press:

The FDA and Worldwide Quality System Requirements Guidebook for Medical Devices, Second Edition
Amiram Daniel and Ed Kimmelman

CAPA for the FDA-Regulated Industry
José Rodríguez-Pérez

Development of FDA-Regulated Medical Products: Prescription Drugs, Biologics, and Medical Devices
Elaine Whitmore

Safe and Sound Software: Creating an Efficient and Effective Quality System for Software Medical Device Organizations
Thomas H. Faris

The Certified Quality Engineer Handbook, Third Edition
Connie M. Borror, editor

Root Cause Analysis: Simplified Tools and Techniques, Second Edition
Bjørn Andersen and Tom Fagerhaug

Mastering and Managing the FDA Maze: Medical Device Overview
Gordon Harnack

Root Cause Analysis: The Core of Problem Solving and Corrective Action
Duke Okes

Get It Right: A Guide to Strategic Quality Systems
Ken Imler

The Internal Auditing Pocket Guide: Preparing, Performing, Reporting, and Follow-up, Second Edition
J.P. Russell

Measurement Matters: How Effective Assessment Drives Business and Safety Performance
Brooks Carder and Patrick Ragan

The Quality Toolbox, Second Edition
Nancy R. Tague

To request a complimentary catalog of ASQ Quality Press publications, call 800-248-1946, or visit our website at www.asq.org/quality-press.

Medical Device Design and Regulation

Carl T. DeMarco

ASQ Quality Press
Milwaukee, Wisconsin

American Society for Quality, Quality Press, Milwaukee 53203
© 2011 by ASQ
All rights reserved. Published 2011
Printed in the United States of America
17 16 15 14 13 12 11   5 4 3 2 1

Library of Congress Cataloging-in-Publication Data

DeMarco, Carl T.
    Medical device design and regulation / Carl T. DeMarco.
        p. cm.
    Includes bibliographical references and index.
    ISBN 978-0-87389-816-4 (hbk. : alk. paper)
    1. Medical instruments and apparatus—United States. 2. Medical instruments
and apparatus—United States—Design and construction. 3. Medical instruments and
apparatus—Safety regulations—United States. 4. Medical instruments and apparatus
industry—United States. I. Title.

    R856.D437 2011
    610.28'4—dc22   2011003881

ISBN: 978-0-87389-816-4

Publisher: William A. Tony
Acquisitions Editor: Matt T. Meinholz
Project Editor: Paul O'Mara
Production Administrator: Randall Benson

ASQ Mission: The American Society for Quality advances individual, organizational,
and community excellence worldwide through learning, quality improvement, and
knowledge exchange.

Attention Bookstores, Wholesalers, Schools, and Corporations: ASQ Quality Press
books, video, audio, and software are available at quantity discounts with bulk
purchases for business, educational, or instructional use. For information, please
contact ASQ Quality Press at 800-248-1946, or write to ASQ Quality Press,
P.O. Box 3005, Milwaukee, WI 53201-3005.

To place orders or to request ASQ membership information, call 800-248-1946. Visit our
website at http://www.asq.org/quality-press.

 Printed on acid-free paper

Quality Press
600 N. Plankinton Ave.
Milwaukee, WI 53203-2914
E-mail: authors@asq.org

The Global Voice of Quality™

This book is dedicated to the many brilliant and creative men and women who labor in the medical device industry and the Food and Drug Administration designing, testing, evaluating, producing, and marketing medical devices for use in the healthcare system for the benefit of mankind.

Table of Contents

List of Figures and Tables

List of Abbreviations

510(k)—Premarket Notification

ADN —annual distribution number

AE —adverse event

AED—automatic external defibrillator

AIP—Application Integrity Policy

ANDA—Abbreviated New Drug Application

ANPRM—Advance Notice of Proposed Rulemaking

ANSI—American National Standards Institute

AP—accredited persons

BIMO —Bioresearch Monitoring Program

BLA —Biologics License Application

CAPA —corrective and preventive action

CBER—Center for Biologics Evaluation and Research

CCI—confidential commercial information

CDC—Centers for Disease Control and Prevention

CDER—Center for Drug Evaluation and Research

CDRH—Center for Devices and Radiological Health

CFG—Certificate for Foreign Government

CFSAN—Center for Food Safety and Applied Nutrition

CGMPs—Current Good Manufacturing Practices

CI—clinical investigator

CMS—Centers for Medicare and Medicaid Services

CRADA—Cooperative Research and Development Agreements

CRFs—case report forms

CRO—contract research organization

CTP—Center for Tobacco Products

CVM—Center for Veterinary Medicine

DHF—design history file

DHHS—U.S. Department of Health and Human Services

DHR—device history record

DMC—data monitoring committee

DMR—device master record

DSMICA—Division of Small Manufacturers, International and Consumer Assistance

EIR—Establishment Inspection Report

eMDR—Electronic Medical Device Reports

EtO—Ethylene Oxide

EU—European Union

FDA—U. S. Food and Drug Administration

FDAAA—Food and Drug Administration Amendments Act of 2007

FDAMA—Food and Drug Administration Modernization Act of 1997

FDCA—Federal Food, Drug, and Cosmetic Act

FEA—finite element analysis

FOIA—Freedom of Information Act

FR—*Federal Register*

GCP—Good clinical practice

GHTF—Global Harmonization Task Force

GLP—Good Laboratory Practice regulation

GLPs—good laboratory practices

GMP—Good Manufacturing Practice regulation

HDE—humanitarian device exemption

HFE—human factors engineering

HHE—Health Hazard Evaluation

HIPAA—Health Insurance Portability and Accountability Act of 1996

HUD—Humanitarian Use Device

IAA—Interagency Agreements

IDE—investigational device exemption

IH—Integrity Hold

IND—investigational new drug

IOM—Institute of Medicine

IRB—institutional review board

ISO—International Standards Organization

JFA—Joint Fellowship Agreement

MDA—Medical Device Amendments of 1976

MDFP—Medical Device Fellowship Program

MDR—Medical Device Reporting regulation

MDRs—Medical Device Reports

MQSA—Mammography Quality Standards Act

MOU—memorandums of understanding

NAI—No Action Indicated

NCTR—National Center for Toxicological Research

NDA—New Drug Application

NGO—nongovernmental organization

NIH—National Institutes of Health

NSE—not substantially equivalent

NSR—nonsignificant risk

OAI—Official Action Indicated

OC—Office of Compliance

OCP—Office of Combination Products

OCER—Office of Communication, Education, and Radiation Programs

ODE—Office of Device Evaluation

OIVD—Office of In Vitro Diagnostic Device Evaluation and Safety

OOPD—Office of Orphan Products Development

ORA—Office of Regulatory Affairs

OSB—Office of Surveillance and Biometrics

OSEL—Office of Science and Engineering Laboratories

OTC—over-the-counter

OUS—outside the United States

PAS—post-approval study

PDP—Product Development Protocol

PHSA—Public Health Service Act

PMA—Premarket Approval

PMR—Postmarketing Requirement

PRS—Protocol Registration System

PS—post-market surveillance

QAU—quality assurance unit

QR—quality system record

QSIT—quality systems inspection technique

QSR—Quality System Regulation

RCHSA—Radiation Control for Health and Safety Act of 1968

RPM—Regulatory Procedures Manual

S&E—safety and effectiveness

SAL—sterility assurance level

SE—substantial equivalence

SGE—special government employee

SMDA—Safe Medical Devices Act of 1990

SOPs—standard operating procedures

SR—significant risk

SSED—Summary of Safety and Effectiveness Data

TRO—temporary restraining order

USC—United States Code

VAI—Voluntary Action Indicated

WL—Warning Letter

WWW—World Wide Web

Introduction

MEDICAL DEVICE REGULATORY REQUIREMENTS

The designing, testing, manufacturing, and marketing of a medical device represent a tremendous scientific, engineering, medical, and business undertaking. There is, however, another, ancillary dimension to such an endeavor that may not always be considered or understood by those entering and practicing in the field of medical devices. Every step in this process is subject to a myriad of complex and specific rules and regulations. These requirements contribute to the precision of the functions that have to be fulfilled in the production of a medical device. Failure to abide by these regulatory requirements can have a devastating effect on the outcome of this effort, and it can end up being extremely costly and time-consuming. Hopefully, the materials presented in this book will create an awareness of these requirements and contribute to an efficient and effective realization of the underlying reason for developing a medical device: to bring to the patient care system a safe and effective device of high quality for the diagnosis or treatment of a human disease or condition.

PURPOSE OF *MEDICAL DEVICE DESIGN AND REGULATION*

The intent of *Medical Device Design and Regulation (MDDR)* is to present an introduction to, and overview of, the world of medical device regulation by the United States Food and Drug Administration (FDA) and the relationship of this regulatory scheme to the design and development of medical devices. This regulatory milieu can be thought of as a culture medium for medical devices. The devices enter this system at the time of design, then grow and mature until they are ready for marketing and use in the healthcare system. In providing this information, the book covers the broad range of requirements, which are presented within eight major topics: background and regulatory environment, device design control, nonclinical testing, clinical trials, marketing applications, post-market requirements, quality systems/GMPs, and compliance/enforcement.

In preparing the materials presented in *MDDR,* there were a series of difficult decisions that had to be made, that is, what information should be included or excluded from the text in a book of such broad scope. Fortunately, during my many years at FDA I had the occasion to interact with many industry executives and their lawyers and consultants. I have discussed industry and company "viewpoints," and I had to explain, in countless discussions and communications, the requirements that had to be met and how to do so. This experience was invaluable in making these inclusion and exclusion decisions so that *MDDR* covers what I perceive industry professionals need to be aware of concerning the regulatory system for medical devices.

This book is not intended to be a "how to" guide, and it does not contain step-by-step instructions on solving specific regulatory issues. *MDDR* provides students and professionals in the medical device industry with a road map to the regulation of medical devices. This textbook, instead of looking in detail at a particular tree, describes the forest into which the uninitiated are entering. It will provide a broad understanding of the breadth and depth of medical device regulation.

There are many specialized books and articles that delve deeply into the individual topics covered in this text. *MDDR* makes a contribution by collecting in one textbook broad coverage of the regulatory scheme for medical devices in terms that are suitable for engineers, scientists, and healthcare providers. This textbook distills from the thousands and thousands of available pages a concise and coherent presentation of this vast amount of information on the subject. Hopefully, the information presented here and the pointers provided will alleviate some of the difficulties that might be encountered by a layperson wanting to find applicable information on medical device regulation. *MDDR* provides a summary of this information and can serve as a road map to more detailed information if desired. In this sense, *MDDR* can serve either as a textbook or a bookshelf reference.

For those wishing more specialized information on a particular topic, there are many continuing education courses regularly offered that provide how-to knowledge about the topics presented here. Attending such CE courses and exploring the literature should satisfy most needs. If that is not sufficient, then it may be necessary to seek professional advice from a regulatory affairs specialist or a medical device lawyer. For designers of innovative medical devices who need a definitive answer concerning a specific issue or issues that arise during the development process it may be necessary to consult with CDRH. This is especially true for innovative device technologies that raise new questions concerning topics such as the appropriate animal model to use in testing, the number of subjects or sites for a clinical trial, the type of statistical analysis that will be acceptable, the specific wording of an informed consent form, and many other issues that can arise during the device development process. For answers to these kinds of questions, it may be necessary to consult with the appropriate review division within the CDRH. *MDDR* repeats this advice in multiple places throughout the text.

FDA's decision-making process is described throughout the book. It is presented in the discussion of agency procedures and actions taken by FDA. When appropriate, the text identifies organizational structures that are involved in various decisions and the factors that are considered in making review decisions. The process is further illustrated by the excerpts from FDA Warning Letters and recall notices and in the cited regulatory and guidance documents. Anyone who reads *MDDR* should have a very good idea about how FDA makes its decisions.

It also should be pointed out that *MDDR*, as a textbook and reference, is not designed to follow current events. It would not be practical to try to describe every specific change FDA makes in response to current conditions. For example, from time to time FDA changes its review and compliance objectives and the resources allocated to these activities. This is discussed in the first chapter under FDA Decision Making where it states, in part:

> The second major balancing act the agency and CDRH must accomplish is the distribution of its finite resources between premarket evaluation and post-market surveillance, including compliance activities. Allocating more resources to premarket evaluation can result in reduced review times for premarket applications, resulting in products arriving sooner in the marketplace for application in patient care. Applying more resources to post-market surveillance and compliance will result in a greater assurance that marketed products continue to provide the intended benefit with the lowest risk of injury or harm to users. The balance between premarket review and post-market surveillance may change from time to time depending on the public health need of the

community for new and better devices versus the need to enhance the protection of users from the risks presented by devices already in the marketplace.

It would not be possible to track every specific change FDA makes in response to current conditions. That function is served by newsletters and journals on a regular basis.

STUDENTS

The book is based on the course I teach to senior and graduate biomedical engineering students at the Engineering School at the Catholic University of America in Washington, D.C., under the department chairmanship of Dr. Binh Tranh. A course like this is generally not taught in engineering schools even though some of their students, especially those undertaking a biomedical engineering major, plan on entering practice in the medical device industry. These students are mostly clueless on how medical devices are regulated and how such regulatory requirements will affect their future professional practice. The availability of this textbook may encourage the offering of such a course in the appropriate college curriculum, especially in engineering schools where the students are known to be planning a career in the medical device industry.

MEDICAL DEVICE PRACTITIONERS

Generally, engineers, scientists, and healthcare practitioners going to work in the medical device industry have not been formally introduced to the regulation of medical devices. They are not offered a course in medical device regulation during their professional education. Most of them embark on a career in the medical device industry with a sound basis in the sciences but without an adequate understanding of the regulatory requirements that will govern their every activity in the design, development, and use of a medical device.

This view was confirmed during my many years of work at FDA, during which time I had numerous occasions to deal with violative firms. Lack of training on FDA requirements was almost always one of the underlying factors contributing to the violative conduct. That is why FDA frequently requires initial and periodic training of company employees on FDA requirements as part of a company's corrective and preventive action plan.

Some medical device manufacturers recognize this need and provide new-employee training in this area. This book can help fill that void. *MDDR* may serve as an aid for device manufacturers and other regulated entities in the introductory training of recently hired employees. It should help give these new practitioners a broad understanding and appreciation of the care that must be exercised as they perform their professional duties within the establishment. It also will help them understand the interrelationship between the various functions being performed within the organization.

MDDR may even appeal to veteran professionals with years of experience in the industry because it will provide information about areas of regulation in which they may not have been active. For example, an employee that has been working for many years in manufacturing may not know much about the requirements related to clinical trials. Another employee that has been involved in the preparation of 510(k)s may know very little about the requirements of a premarket approval (PMA) application. In other words, years of experience do not guarantee that an individual has the breadth of knowledge that is presented in this text.

As stated before, the content of *MDDR* is just a starting point, but an important one because it provides the scope and layout of the regulatory scheme. It is left to the reader to acquire more in-depth knowledge, as necessary, depending on the functions being performed. *MDDR* provides the pointers to these additional sources of more-detailed information.

DEVICE DESIGN AND INNOVATION

Device design and innovation is a process that may extend throughout the testing, manufacturing, and marketing of a medical device. Information or events that arise after the initial design work is completed may necessitate the return to the design stage to make compensating changes in the original design. This can occur during the manufacturing process or during the post-market experience with the device. It may occur because of the discovery of a device defect during testing or manufacturing, the receipt of consumer or user complaints, the need for a recall, or the receipt of a Warning Letter from FDA. The information that appears in the chapters beyond Chapter 2, Medical Device Design, deal with these other factors that may arise throughout the life cycle of a medical device. An awareness of these implications is important for those involved in the design of a new or innovative device because they may affect the design of the device and ultimately require design changes.

A RISK-BASED REGULATORY SYSTEM

Medical devices are an essential component of healthcare. They provide a valuable resource in the diagnosis, treatment, and cure of disease in humans. However, the use of medical devices also presents a wide range of risks to patients and users. Some risks are minor and easily dealt with while others may involve serious injury and even death.

In order to safely bring the many benefits of medical device technology to patients around the world, the Congress of the United States adopted, and U.S. Food and Drug Administration administers, a risk-based system for the regulation of medical devices. Devices that present the lowest risk to patients and users are subject to the lowest level of regulation while the highest-risk devices must meet the most rigorous level of scrutiny and control.

This risk-based system is discussed directly under the classification of medical devices in Chapter 1, part 13, Medical Devices, Drugs, and Biologics. The different regulatory requirements for devices with differing levels of risk will also be apparent in the discussion of many topics throughout the text.

INTERNATIONAL ASPECTS OF MEDICAL DEVICE REGULATION

Many nations have some form of regulation for medical devices. The more developed nations have more-sophisticated regulatory systems while the developing countries have relatively simplified systems. The laws and regulations of countries outside the United States are beyond the scope of this book because of the extent, variety, and complexity of those laws and regulations. However, the following summary information related to commerce in medical devices between the United States and other nations may be of interest to readers.

Chapter 1, part 9, section 1, European Union Medical Device Regulation, provides a brief overview of the system for regulation of medical devices in the European Union, and section 2, Global Harmonization Task Force, discusses the international efforts to reconcile the regulatory requirements of various countries to minimize the burden of differing requirements on international commerce. Chapter 4, part 1, section 2, International Guidelines for Medical Devices Research, discusses the gathering of human test data outside of the United States. Chapter 4, part 7, Importing and Exporting Medical Devices for Investigational Use, covers the import and export of investigational medical devices. Chapter 5, part 1, section 2, Valid Scientific Evidence, explains the use of foreign research data in marketing applications. Chapter 5, part 4, Importing and Exporting

Medical Devices for Commercial Distribution deals with the import or export of medical devices for marketing purposes. Lastly, Chapter 1, part 5, Quasi-Legal Requirements, explores the application of consensus standards developed by international organizations.

LEARNING AIDES

The text contains several aids to make it easier to navigate this body of information and to more quickly find the required information. In addition to an index, the table of contents identifies chapters, parts, and sections so the reader can easily find the sought-after information. This expanded table of contents also shows the relationship of each topic to other topics in the greater scheme of information.

A great deal of the information presented in the text, such as regulations, guidances, standards, and *Federal Register* documents, is illustrated through the inclusion of numerous quotes from FDA Warning Letters and recall notices that demonstrate FDA's thinking on the topic and the application of various requirements to practices encountered in company actions.

There is a great deal of information available for free on the Internet. Most of the information about the regulatory scheme for medical devices resides on the FDA website. That is why *MDDR* contains over 100 links to Internet sites, primarily FDA's web pages, which contain more in-depth information on the topics being discussed. These links serve several purposes. Importantly, *MDDR* saves the reader time in finding relevant information on a particular topic. Secondly, it provides the reader access to more-detailed information on each of the topics discussed in *MDDR*. This is important because only so much information can be presented in a textbook that is presenting an overview of the medical device regulatory scheme. The third benefit is to provide familiarity with the FDA website. For a professional in the medical device field it is critical to understand FDA's policies and practices, many of which are found on the FDA website, in order to successfully navigate the regulatory system to obtain a successful outcome in dealing with the agency.

Last but not least, these citations will lead to the latest versions of regulations, guidances, and standards related to medical devices. Regulations, standards, and guidance documents undergo regular review and revision. For example, some standards organizations stipulate that their standards be reviewed and updated every five years. Sometimes they are updated before five years have elapsed when the need arises. That is particularly true for the newer standards. The same holds true for FDA regulations and guidances. Therefore, it is important to make sure you are using the current versions of these documents by checking the appropriate website.

The live hyperlinks to these websites are collected in Appendix A, which is available in electronic format containing live hyperlinks for easy access to the web pages cited in the text. This electronic version is being provided on a CD, which can be found inside the back cover. It may also be obtained via free download from the American Society for Quality (ASQ) website at http://asq.org/, or by e-mailing authors@asq.org. The CD or the downloaded appendix will allow a direct link to each of the listed websites, thus eliminating the need to type lengthy URLs in order to reach the desired web page.

Over time, the FDA's website and some of its citations may change. If the included citation does not yield the expected page, it is advisable to use appropriate search terms to locate the desired document.

There also are problems and projects at the end of each chapter that will enable the student or reader to test their knowledge and understanding of the materials presented in that chapter. In addition to the usual questions requiring specific answers, the projects include the drafting of a device control plan, the development of a nonclinical test procedure, the resolution of a recall, the response to a Warning Letter, and the creation of a CAPA for a device deficiency. A solutions manual for these exercises is available to teachers who adopt the textbook for classroom use.

Lastly, owners of *MDDR* may join the "MDDR Users Group" on LinkedIn by e-mailing authors@asq.org. The *MDDR* Users Group will provide a forum for readers to exchange ideas, share experiences, and seek advice from other users. The author will also be a member and participate from time to time.

FIELD TESTING

As stated above, the materials in this book have been "field tested" in the classroom in a graduate seminar at the Engineering School at the Catholic University of America. The materials in this book come largely from my lecture notes and classroom discussions. It also includes some information gleaned from the presentations of guest lecturers who are experts in the areas of their presentations. The guest lecturers included the following individuals:

Edward Basile, BME, JD
Senior Partner
King & Spalding
700 Pennsylvania Avenue, NW, Suite 200
Washington, DC 20006-4706

Peter Carstensen, BME
Senior Analyst
Wiklund Research & Design
152 Commonwealth Avenue
Concord, MA 01742

Christy Foreman, BSBME, MBE
Deputy Director and Acting Director
Office of Device Evaluation
Center for Devices and Radiological Health
10903 New Hampshire Avenue
Silver Spring, MD 20993

Jonette Foy, BME, PhD
Chief, Orthopedic Joint Devices Branch
and Acting Deputy Director, Office of Device Evaluation
Center for Devices and Radiological Health
10903 New Hampshire Avenue
Silver Spring, MD 20993

Michael Marcarelli, MS, PharmD
Director, Division of Bioresearch Monitoring
Center for Devices and Radiological Health
10903 New Hampshire Avenue
Silver Spring, MD 20993

Larry R. Pilot, BS Pharm, JD
McKenna Long & Aldridge LLP
1900 K Street NW
Washington, DC 20006-1108

Miriam Provost, PhD
Senior Consultant, Medical Devices
Biologics Consulting Group, Inc.
400 N. Washington Street, Suite 100
Alexandria, VA 22314

Donna Bea Tillman, BSE, PhD
Former Director
Office of Device Evaluation
Center for Devices and Radiological Health
10903 New Hampshire Avenue
Silver Spring, MD 20993

David L. West, PhD, MPH
Vice President, Medical Device Development

Quintiles
1801 Rockville Pike, Suite 300
Rockville, MD 20852

Lynette Zentgraft, BSBME, MS
Regulatory Submissions and Strategy Expert
King & Spalding
1700 Pennsylvania Avenue, NW, Suite 200
Washington, DC 20006-4706

It is important to point out that the guest lecturers appeared in their personal capacity and not as representatives of their respective employers, and their presentations represented their personal views and did not necessarily represent the views of their employers.

CAVEATS

All of the information in *MDDR,* including the websites and other references in the text, was current when the text was prepared. However, all of these references are subject to revision whenever it is deemed necessary by the agency or sponsoring organization. It is necessary to keep up to date on the rapid changes occurring in the field of medical devices. For example, see the discussions under Chapter 1, part 3, section 3, CDRH Strategic Priorities and Transparency, and Chapter 5, part 2, section 9, Upcoming 510(k) Program Changes. Current developments should be monitored through the trade press, the professional literature, and the FDA website to determine any effect subsequent changes might have on day-to-day practices.

Device design, nonclinical testing, and clinical trials are discussed in Chapters 2 through 4. However, the outcomes of these tasks will be used in marketing applications for approval or clearance. Therefore, it will be useful to read the corresponding discussions of these topics as they are presented in Chapter 5, Marketing Applications, which elaborate on how FDA will evaluate the resulting data and information in evaluating an application.

DISCLAIMER

This text will not make a regulatory expert out of the reader, nor is it intended to provide legal advice on any specific issue or controversy that may arise. If a serious legal or regulatory problem arises, the reader is advised to seek the advice of a competent consultant or legal counsel. Failure to do so may result in undesirable civil or criminal consequences.

Acknowledgments

First, I wish to acknowledge Dr. Binh Tranh's foresight in offering my seminar to the biomedical engineering students at the Catholic University of America. This course convinced me that a textbook like *MDDR* could make a contribution to those who were involved in the design of medical devices.

Next, I want to express my deep appreciation to the guest lecturers listed in the Introduction whose outstanding presentations enriched the learning experience for the students in my classes. The students, likewise, expressed their profound appreciation for the lectures presented by the guest speakers.

I wish to also gratefully acknowledge the time devoted by the following experts who conducted a substantive review of all or parts of the manuscript and provided cogent comments on the text:

Peter Carstensen, BME
Senior Analyst
Wiklund Research & Design

Christy Foreman, BSBME, MBE
Deputy Director and Acting Director
Office of Device Evaluation
Center for Devices and Radiological Health

David L. West, PhD, MPH
Vice President, Medical Device Development
Quintiles

Lastly, I want to acknowledge the time and effort of Dan DeMarco and Angela DeMarco, who fastidiously and expertly edited this manuscript.

1

Background and Regulatory Environment

This chapter of the book provides basic background information on the design and development of a medical device, the medical device industry, the Food and Drug Administration, and the legal and regulatory environment applicable to medical devices. In this scenario, FDA is the regulating party, and the medical device industry in all of its permutations is the regulated party. Within this relationship, each party has rights and duties or obligations that are imposed by law. These rights and duties define the conduct of each party and determine what either party may or may not do.

The Federal Food, Drug, and Cosmetic Act (FDCA) provides the basic framework for the industry–FDA relationship. However, there is a plethora of other laws and regulations that govern their interactions as well. The United States Constitution provides the underpinning of our legal system. Within the system affecting this relationship, in addition to constitutional prescriptions and the FDCA, there are laws related to the administrative process, the criminal code, and decisional law emanating from the judicial system. The focus of this book is on the FDCA and FDA regulations, and these collateral requirements are considered as needed to round out the topics under discussion.

Also included in this chapter are topics that are universal in their applicability and not related to just one area of medical device design and development. For example, this chapter includes discussions of patents, confidentiality of nonpublic information, monitoring and auditing, and international aspects of device regulation.

PART 1. MEDICAL DEVICE DESIGN AND DEVELOPMENT

The design and development of a medical device involves a great deal of complex decision making. Consideration must be given to the needs of individual patients and the healthcare system, the requirements of the business model being used, the financial aspects of the undertaking, pricing and reimbursement, scientific and medical issues, regulatory requirements, applicable standards, manufacturing quality into the device, and marketing strategies, to name just some areas of concern.

Medical device design and development has evolved from the use of intuition, creativity, and trial and error to the present methodology in which devices are developed under a disciplined "quality system" subject to regulation and measured against the requirements of laws, regulations, and national standards. In addition, internationally recognized concepts of design control and quality systems applied to the development of a medical device now greatly impact how the device will be accepted for marketing in the United States, European Union, and emerging markets. Thus, devices developed employing these concepts will more readily meet requirements in global markets. Moreover, disciplined development will help address strategies and data requirements for reimbursement and help protect against personal injury litigation.

Section 1. Major Steps in the Design and Development of a Medical Device

As stated in the introduction, the continuum from the concept of a medical device to its eventual marketing and use in healthcare can be segmented in various ways. For the purpose of this book, the following major steps are used as a guide to the development of a medical device. The various responsibilities and obligations that attach to these steps will be discussed throughout the text.

1. *Medical device design.* There are very few regulatory responsibilities that attach to the conceptual work and basic research involved in medical device design. FDA regulation comes into play when the developer moves out of the realm of research and into the realm of development by committing itself to the development of a specific device. Medical device design activities to implement the concept of the device are discussed in Chapter 2.

2. *Nonclinical testing.* Nonclinical testing of prototypes and the finished device, which would include laboratory testing and animal testing, is covered in Chapter 3. This chapter includes a discussion of Good Laboratory Practices, which is a set of regulations that provide requirements on the design, conduct, and documentation of the testing.

3. *Clinical trials.* Chapter 4 deals with clinical studies of the device in human subjects.

4. *Marketing applications.* The premarket applications and their evaluation necessary to obtain marketing approval are discussed in Chapter 5.

5. *Post-approval requirements.* Chapter 6 discusses the continuing post-approval responsibilities of manufacturers after the device is placed into commercial distribution for medical use.

6. *Manufacturing.* Manufacturing the device for marketing under the Quality System Regulation is examined in Chapter 7.

7. *Compliance and enforcement.* Chapter 8 examines compliance and enforcement actions that are available to FDA when there are violations of the legal and regulatory requirements of the Food, Drug, and Cosmetic Act and FDA regulations.

Section 2. Teamwork in Industry and FDA

In the industry and at FDA, teamwork is an important factor in the design, development, and evaluation of a medical device. While there may be examples of an individual working alone in the "garage" developing a medical device, such creativity would be an exceptional occurrence. Most often, the development of a medical device requires the creative genius of a variety of individuals, frequently with different expertise.

The same is true for the review and evaluation of submissions by FDA. Teams of individuals with varied but necessary expertise are utilized by the agency to assure complete and accurate assessments of pending submissions and potential enforcement actions.

The following list identifies some of the types of experts that may be involved in the development and regulation of a medical device, depending on the intended use of the device, its design, functions, materials, and components:

- *Engineers.* Engineers are almost always involved in medical device design, especially biomedical and mechanical engineers. Electrical, software, and other engineers may also be needed depending on the device under development. Engineers are also critical when it comes time to transfer the device design to the manufacturing stage and in reviewing and analyzing complaints about malfunction of the device.

- *Chemists.* Various types of chemists and chemical engineers may be needed in the design and development of a medical device, especially if plastics, organic matrices, metals, or exotic chemical-based substances are part of the device.

- *Biologists/physiologists/microbiologists/anatomists.* Professionals with expertise in the biological sciences may be needed in the design of a device, depending on its intended use, and especially during the different testing stages of the device, including both animal and clinical testing.

- *Physicians, nurses, and healthcare practitioners.* These healthcare providers, and others such as physical and occupational therapists, have a role to play in the design and clinical testing of medical devices. Their experience in patient care is essential during the design stage, in clinical testing, and when creating adequate instructions for use.

- *Statisticians.* Statisticians, especially biostatisticians, are frequently essential in the design of laboratory and clinical testing and in data analysis.

Hopefully, these professionals will benefit from the information and guidance in this book. The reader should keep in mind, however, that this book will not make one an expert in medical device laws and regulations. To maintain current knowledge and skills during practice, professionals in the field of medical device design and development regularly attend in-depth continuing education courses on medical device laws and regulations pertaining to their particular area of practice. This practice is highly recommended for active professionals.

Section 3. Medical Device Quality, Safety, and Effectiveness

The medical device industry and the FDA, along with regulatory bodies throughout the world, share a mutual goal of bringing to the healthcare

Table 1.1 Pillars of the FDA regulatory scheme to assure quality, safety, and effectiveness.

Premarket	Post-market
Design control	Good manufacturing practices
Nonclinical testing	Quality systems inspection technique (QSIT) inspections
Clinical testing	Post-market studies
Bioresearch monitoring	Post-market surveillance and reporting
Premarket review	Notification/3Rs
Labeling	Recalls
Good manufacturing practices	Corrective and preventive action (CAPA)

system medical devices that are of a high quality and that are safe and effective for their intended uses. Without the cooperation of both parties, this goal would be more difficult to achieve.

The industry and FDA both know of the activities that, if executed properly, further the goal of globally delivering safe, effective, and high-quality devices to healthcare providers and their patients. The FDA regulatory scheme rests on two primary pillars that monitor and regulate these activities (see Table 1.1). These pillars are supported by the law and FDA implementing regulations, FDA guidance documents, scientific laboratories, and enforcement actions.

PART 2. THE MEDICAL DEVICE INDUSTRY

We would not have medical devices without a medical device industry. The "medical device industry" is generally considered to be the companies that actually design, manufacture, and market medical devices. This would include those who develop specifications for medical devices and those companies that actually produce and initially market the products. The heaviest regulatory burdens under the FDCA and FDA regulations fall upon this sector.

Section 1. Industry Demographics

The medical device industry is a major component of the U.S. economy. According to an FDA count as of June 24, 2010, there were 7748 domestic firms listed in the Center for Devices and Radiological Health (CDRH) establishment registration and device listing database. According to the Advanced Medical Technology Association (AdvaMed), a major industry trade association, they employ over 357,000 employees paying out some $22 billion in salaries. California has the largest number of jobs in the industry with 72,500 workers, followed by Massachusetts, Florida, Minnesota, New Jersey, and Pennsylvania.

Despite the size of the industry, 90% of the manufacturers in the United States have fewer than 100 employees, and 80% of the device manufacturers in the United States have sales of less than $30 million.

In the large majority of states, salary rates for the industry are above the state average because it requires a highly skilled workforce. Medical technology jobs pay an average of 30% more than the average job, and each medical technology job generates 4.5 additional jobs from suppliers.

Section 2. Medical Device Innovations

The medical device industry is a high-tech industry. Every year, the industry markets new devices that represent major steps forward in the advancement of patient care. These devices are used in the diagnosis, treatment, and cure of diseases, employing the latest scientific developments. The trends in the use of new technologies in medical devices include computer-related systems, telemedicine, wireless systems, robotics, new energy sources, molecular medicine, nanotechnology, new materials, minimally invasive instrumentation, and organ and tissue replacements.

Devices are in development long before they are discussed with FDA at pre-submission meetings, and even longer before they are actually approved or cleared for marketing. These innovations in medical device design are advancing the various areas of medicine and can be found in discussions presented in the current scientific and engineering journal articles, in the trade press, and in financial and investment reports.

Section 3. The Regulated Industry

The term *regulated industry*, as opposed to the term *medical device industry*, refers to more than just manufacturers of medical devices, and encompasses a much broader spectrum of persons dealing with medical devices. It includes—in relationship to medical devices—importers, distributors, and other sellers of medical devices. It extends to user facilities such as hospitals, extended care facilities, and nursing homes using medical devices in the provision of healthcare services, physicians, clinics, and other professional providers conducting clinical trials. It even encompasses other government agencies, such as NIH, performing research and other functions related to medical devices. All of these parties, in addition to the medical device industry, are regulated to varying degrees by FDA depending on their activities, and are included in the discussion of various topics as necessary throughout the book.

PART 3. UNITED STATES FOOD AND DRUG ADMINISTRATION

Section 1. Organizational Structure

United States Department of Health and Human Services

The United States Food and Drug Administration (FDA) resides in the United States Department of Health and Human Services (DHHS) along with its sister agencies such as the National Institutes of Health (NIH), the Centers for Disease Control and Prevention (CDC), and an alphabet soup of others (see Figure 1.1).

The Food and Drug Administration

The FDA is a large federal agency with over 10,000 employees nationwide. FDA has many responsibilities. The major FDA goals, as dealt with in this book, are to ensure that medical devices are safe and effective, that safe and effective products are efficiently delivered to patients, that these products are of sufficient quality and perform as claimed, and that medical claims are supported by valid scientific evidence. The FDA is composed of several major operating units. The main one of concern in the

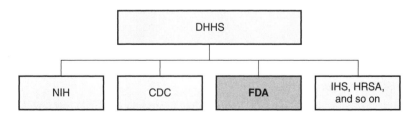

Figure 1.1   DHHS organization chart.

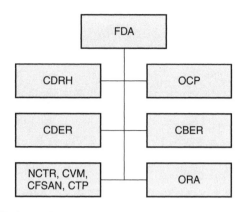

Figure 1.2 FDA organization chart.

area of medical devices is the Center for Devices and Radiological Health (CDRH), along with the Center for Drug Evaluation and Research (CDER), the Center for Biologics Evaluation and Research (CBER), the Office of Combination Products (OCP), and the Office of Regulatory Affairs (ORA). The agency also includes the National Center for Toxicological Research (NCTR), the Center for Veterinary Medicine (CVM), the Center for Food Safety and Applied Nutrition (CFSAN), and the newly formed Center for Tobacco Products (CTP) as set forth in Figure 1.2.

The Center for Devices and Radiological Health

The CDRH is the center within FDA that is directly responsible for the medical device program. CDRH has over 1000 dedicated, highly skilled, and internationally respected public health employees and comprises the major operating units depicted in Figure 1.3. These offices are described below. There are also several support units not displayed in Figure 1.3 dealing with management operations and post-market transformation, and a CDRH ombudsman.

The following is a brief description of the mission statement of CDRH and its major operating units. These offices and their program activities are discussed in more detail, as necessary, elsewhere in the book in relation to the topics under consideration.

CDRH Responsibilities

In the broadest sense, CDRH is responsible for regulating firms who manufacture, repackage, relabel, or import medical devices sold in the United States. In addition, CDRH regulates radiation-emitting electronic products

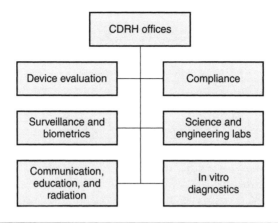

Figure 1.3   CDRH organization chart.

(medical and nonmedical) such as lasers, x-ray systems, ultrasound equipment, microwave ovens, and color televisions. The Center comprises, and accomplishes its mission through, the following major operating offices.

Office of Device Evaluation (ODE)

ODE is responsible for the program areas through which medical devices are evaluated or cleared for clinical trials and marketing. The major programs administered by ODE include premarket approval, product development protocol, humanitarian device exemption, investigational device exemption, and premarket notification programs.

Office of Surveillance and Biometrics (OSB)

OSB is responsible for monitoring the continued safety and effectiveness of medical devices after they have reached the marketplace. OSB also provides statistical and epidemiologic expertise in market approval decisions made by the Center. OSB conducts statistical analyses, designs and performs targeted epidemiological studies, directs a nationwide surveillance system designed to monitor the performance of marketed medical devices, facilitates cross-Center response when a problem is identified, and provides statistical analyses of studies conducted for the premarket approval process and post-market device performance.

Office of Compliance (OC)

OC has the primary responsibility for enforcing the Federal Food, Drug, and Cosmetic Act and its implementing regulations. It accomplishes its goals through program functions such as registration and listing, recalls, export certificates, and liaison with the Office of Regulatory Affairs and their district offices. Additional program functions include import/export, promotion and advertising, labeling, training, and risk management.

Office of Science and Engineering Laboratories (OSEL)

OSEL is the laboratory of CDRH. OSEL performs product testing, develops reliable standardized test methods for CDRH and industry use, performs anticipatory scientific investigations on emerging technologies, contributes laboratory data to national and international standards used in Center decision making, provides scientific and technical training for CDRH staff members, and maintains laboratory collaborations and relationships with scientific researchers in academia and other federal laboratories. OSEL also coordinates and oversees CDRH's activities that support the development of national and international standards.

Office of Communication, Education, and Radiation Programs (OCER)

OCER supports CDRH in assuring the safety and effectiveness of medical devices and radiation-emitting electronic products by communicating risk and benefit information about these products to the public and educating manufacturers about FDA regulations and policies. OCER also manages the CDRH Radiological Health Program, including the Mammography Quality Standards Act (MQSA).

Office of In Vitro Diagnostic Device Evaluation and Safety (OIVD)

OIVD regulates all aspects of in-home and laboratory diagnostic tests (in vitro diagnostic devices, or IVDs). OIVD combines the functions of other offices within CDRH into one organizational unit by combining the premarket review responsibilities of the ODE, the enforcement responsibilities of the OC, and the post-market surveillance responsibilities of the OSB. OIVD maintains collaborative ties to OSEL for technical assistance and OCER for communication and outreach assistance.

Section 2. FDA Decision Making

In addition to fostering medical device innovation, one of FDA's missions is to get safe and effective devices to market expeditiously while ensuring that the devices on the market remain safe and effective. It accomplishes this primarily through the Center for Devices and Radiological Health. In doing so, CDRH engages in several balancing acts in order to assure that it meets its goals.

The first FDA balancing act is to weigh the benefits and the risks of each device it evaluates. The benefits must outweigh the risks before it will approve a device for marketing. There is no magic end point in making this determination. The agency uses scientific data, inputs from internal and external experts, and the needs of the healthcare system in exercising its judgment on whether a particular device should be marketed.

The second major balancing act the agency and CDRH must accomplish is the distribution of its finite resources between premarket evaluation and post-market surveillance and compliance activities. Allocating more resources to premarket evaluation can result in reduced review times for premarket applications, resulting in products arriving sooner in the marketplace for application in patient care. Applying more resources to post-market surveillance and compliance will result in a greater assurance that marketed products continue to provide the intended benefit with the lowest risk of injury or harm to users. The balance between premarket review and post-market surveillance may change from time to time depending on the public health need of the community for new and better devices versus the need to enhance the protection of users from the risks presented by devices already in the marketplace.

These decisions are very often influenced by outside forces such as congressional oversight activities, the press, and private and public interest groups. The balance of these allocations may change from time to time depending on the magnitude of these influences.

To attack this problem of premarket and post-market needs, CDRH has developed a construct called the *Total Product Life Cycle* approach. This approach is intended to focus attention on the full extent of the use of a device from evolution to final dissipation. The process of moving from conceptualization to development and marketing leads back to new concepts, and so the cycle is self-perpetuating. At all stages of the cycle, FDA seeks to assure the safe and effective use of medical devices available to the American public.

Section 3. CDRH Strategic Priorities and Transparency

Strategic Priorities

As stated in the introduction, the agency's regulations and policies are always subject to change. In January 2010 CDRH published its strategic priorities for review and modification of its regulations and programs. It is important for anyone practicing in the medical device industry to monitor the changes that will take place in the coming months and years. These changes will affect the premarket review programs, compliance programs, communication with the public, and internal management practices. As examples of changes that will be forthcoming, modifications can be expected in the following areas, as well as many other areas of the medical device program:

- Strengthening the 510(k) program and structuring the review of 510(k)s

- Improving the quality of clinical data submitted in support of premarket approvals (PMAs)

- Issuing guidance on study design for clinical trials

- Putting in place systems and procedures to more efficiently and effectively capture, analyze, and share high-quality information about adverse events

- Improving internal processes that relate to personnel, management, information sharing, and so on, to produce more timely and effective decision making

The strategic priorities plan is large and complex. To keep the public informed of developments under this plan, the Center has established a website that identifies the priorities and tracks the progress being made in the implementation of the plan. This information is important to all professionals involved in the design, testing, manufacturing, and marketing of medical devices. It may be accessed at the following web pages:

> http://www.fda.gov/AboutFDA/CentersOffices/CDRH/CDRH VisionandMission/ucm197647.htm

> http://www.fda.gov/AboutFDA/CentersOffices/CDRH/CDRH VisionandMission/ucm232531.htm

Center Transparency

This is one of the critical aspects of FDA's strategic priorities that constitutes a major effort to help consumers, stakeholders, and others understand how the agency operates and makes decisions. The agency formed a Transparency Task Force, which announced the release of 21 draft proposals for public comment on public disclosure policies. The Transparency Task Force will review the comments and decide which proposals to recommend for implementation. In announcing the proposals, the agency stated, "These proposals reflect a careful balancing of the importance of transparency with the importance of protecting trade secrets and confidentiality." The proposals reflect the review of more than 1500 public comments received by the FDA after two public meetings held by the task force, and extensive consideration and discussion within the agency. FDA has made various documents related to this effort available, which may be viewed on the FDA Transparency Task Force home page at:

http://www.fda.gov/AboutFDA/WhatWeDo/FDATransparency TaskForce/default.htm

In support of this new transparency effort, CDRH now posts summaries of internal premarket review memos for 180-day PMA supplements. The agency will soon begin posting decision memos on 510(k)s as well. This is a very important development because it will give the industry and public additional insight into the agency's decision making.

Section 4. Division of Small Manufacturers, International and Consumer Assistance

The Division of Small Manufacturers, International and Consumer Assistance (DSMICA) is a division within CDRH that deserves special identification because of the broad role it plays in the dissemination of information about the regulatory scheme for medical devices. DSMICA is a good place to start within CDRH when seeking information about the medical device programs administered by the agency.

DSMICA provides technical and regulatory information to small manufacturers and others to help them comply with FDA requirements for medical devices. The assistance includes information about product classification, premarket and post-market requirements, labeling, manufacturing requirements (quality system), and import/export issues for medical devices and reporting requirements for electronic products. The division also provides information to consumers regarding medical devices and radiation-emitting products to enhance their ability to avoid risk, achieve maximum benefit, and make informed decisions about the use of such products. Lastly, DSMICA identifies and supports global harmonization activities, educates foreign governments on the United States medical device regulatory process, and directs U.S. firms to sources of information on foreign requirements for medical devices. DSMICA's home page on the FDA website can be found at:

http://www.fda.gov/medicaldevices/deviceregulationand guidance/ucm142656.htm

Section 5. FDA Foreign Offices

The FDA is in the process of establishing offices in foreign countries. FDA's China Office in Beijing is FDA's first foreign location. There will also be secondary offices in Guangzhou and Shanghai. The China offices will be staffed by senior inspectors and senior technical experts in foods, medicines, and medical devices.

According to FDA, "A permanent FDA presence in China will help us address the challenges presented by globalization. We look forward to working with the Chinese government and manufacturers to ensure that FDA standards for safety and manufacturing quality are met before products ship to the United States." FDA will also assist the Chinese government, as requested, in its ongoing efforts to improve its regulatory systems for exports to help assure product safety, and will work with regulated industry to help assure that those wishing to export their products to the United States fully understand U.S. requirements and expectations.

FDA is also in the final process of standing up the in-country components of its offices in India, Europe, Latin America, and the Middle East.

PART 4. THE LEGAL BASIS FOR DEVICE REGULATION

The legal system that provides for, and affects, the regulation of medical devices is broad and complex. It spans a wide variety of laws, regulations, and judicial decisions. These are legal requirements and can be enforced via civil or criminal actions. In addition to these legal requirements, quasi-legal requirements such as voluntary standards and guidance documents must be taken into account. These are not generally enforceable. This part provides an overview of this system as a context for the topics discussed throughout the book.

Section 1. Interstate Commerce

The regulation of medical devices by the federal government begins with the United States Constitution. The "interstate commerce clause" of the constitution, Article I, Section 8, states in part:

> The Congress shall have power . . .
>   To regulate commerce with foreign nations, and among the several states, and with the Indian tribes;

Medical devices, like drugs, foods, and other products regulated by FDA, are commodities of interstate commerce. Congress used this constitutional provision as the authority under which it enacted a pervasive system for the regulation of medical devices.

Section 2. The Federal Food, Drug, and Cosmetic Act (FDCA) and Its Evolution

Since ancient times, foods and drugs have been subjected to some sort of regulation, usually centered on the weight, measure, or purity of these products. This early regulation was very often provided by guilds and professional groups.

In the United States, the regulation of foods, drugs, devices, and biologics underwent an evolutionary process. The first federal law regulating these products was adopted by the U.S. Congress as the Food and Drugs Act of 1906. This law did not expressly apply to medical devices. Neither did it require premarket testing for safety or effectiveness.

In 1938, more than 100 people died after taking Elixir Sulfanilamide. The elixir was prepared with diethylene glycol, a toxic substance. The Congress then enacted a major overhaul of the 1906 act named the Federal Food, Drug, and Cosmetic Act of 1938. This law, the FDCA, continued prohibiting adulterated or misbranded items from commerce. It added the requirement that drugs be tested adequately to establish their safety for use under the conditions set forth on the label. It also required labels to bear warnings about the habit-forming nature of certain drugs, adequate directions for use, and other precautionary measures. For the first time, the FDCA included devices and cosmetics. However, it did not contain the current regulatory scheme for medical devices.

Section 3. The Medical Device Amendments of 1976

In 1970, a study group on medical devices, chaired by Dr. Theodore Cooper, Director of the National Heart and Lung Institute at NIH, issued a report entitled *Medical Devices: A Legislative Plan* dated September 1970. This "Cooper Report" set the stage and initial justification for the subsequent adoption by Congress of amendments to the FDCA known as the Medical Device Amendments of 1976. Since that time there have been many amendments of the device provisions. Some of the major device amendments to the FDCA include, among others: the Safe Medical Devices Act (1990), the Medical Device Amendments (1992), the Mammography Quality Standards Act (1992), the FDA Modernization Act (1998), the Medical Device User Fee and Modernization Act (2002), and the FDA Amendments Act (2007). An extensive listing with brief descriptions of amendments to the FDCA, including those related to other products regulated by FDA, can be found in FDA's "Regulatory Procedures Manual" of March 2009 at the following link:

http://www.fda.gov/downloads/ICECI/ComplianceManuals/
RegulatoryProceduresManual/UCM074340.pdf

The current FDCA, as amended, can be found and searched at:

http://www.fda.gov/opacom/laws/fdcact/fdctoc.htm

Most of the discussion in this book will center around the medical device requirements of the FDCA and FDA's regulations.

PART 5. QUASI-LEGAL REQUIREMENTS

Quasi-legal requirements, within a legal context, are those conditions that are not enforceable as a law or regulation but are used within the regulatory milieu as tools or means of facilitating fulfillment of FDA requirements and meeting agency expectations. They include such items as voluntary standards, some of which may ultimately be recognized by FDA, FDA guidance documents, advisory opinions, some responses to citizens' petitions, and general agency policies and practices. In the medical device area they are used extensively by industry and the FDA.

Section 1. Voluntary/Consensus Standards

There are nongovernmental organizations (NGOs) that issue voluntary standards for various aspects of medical device design and development, such as:

- Association for the Advancement of Medical Instrumentation (AAMI)

- American National Standards Institute (ANSI)

- ASTM International

- Clinical and Laboratory Standards Institute (CLSI)

- International Electrotechnical Commission (IEC)

- International Organization for Standardization (ISO)

These national and international organizations use panels of experts to develop their standards. These experts come from industry, academia, and government agencies.

For medical device standards, CDRH is actively involved in these national and international processes. It is important to distinguish mandatory standards from voluntary standards. As the name indicates, the former are required by FDA and must be met by the manufacturer while the latter may be adopted and used by the manufacturer on a voluntary basis.

A voluntary standard can deal with any issues related to medical devices such as: the processing, content, and evaluation of regulatory submissions; the design, production, manufacturing, and testing of regulated products; and inspection and enforcement procedures. A standard may provide guidance on the design, testing, and manufacture, or the use and labeling of, a medical device. It may establish what are considered to be acceptable standards in the industry for the function to which it applies. The standards are available, usually for a fee, from the NGO that publishes them, and they are in widespread use within the medical device industry.

Section 2. FDA-Recognized Standards

FDA has the authority to recognize all or parts of voluntary standards. Many of these consensus standards have been developed with the participation of CDRH staff. The agency believes that conformance with an agency-recognized consensus standard can support a reasonable assurance of safety or effectiveness for many applicable aspects of a medical device being evaluated under a premarket approval application. Similarly, information on conformance with a recognized consensus standard in a premarket notification may help establish the substantial equivalence of a new device to a legally marketed predicate device.

Thus, when a submission contains a declaration of conformity to a standard in a premarket submission, FDA will accept that the device meets the requirements of the standard as stated in the submission, and the declaration will, in many cases, eliminate the need to review the actual test data for those aspects of the device addressed by the standard. FDA, however, does retain the right to obtain any information authorized by the applicable statute or regulations, including test data substantiating conformance with a standard. Furthermore, FDA may inspect and audit such test data to confirm conformance to a standard as declared in a submission.

Additional detailed information on the recognition and use of consensus standards in marketing applications can be found in the FDA guidance document at:

http://www.fda.gov/downloads/MedicalDevices/Device
RegulationandGuidance/GuidanceDocuments/ucm077295.pdf

FDA maintains a searchable database of recognized standards, which is updated at least once a year, at:

http://www.accessdata.fda.gov/scripts/cdrh/cfdocs/cfStandards/
search.cfm

Section 3. Mandatory Standards

Manufacturers must comply with mandatory standards if required by FDA. Many mandatory standards, if applicable to a specific class of devices or to a specific device, may be found in the classification regulations as discussed in this chapter, part 13, Medical Devices, Drugs, and Biologics.

Section 4. Guidance Documents

From time to time FDA issues guidance documents to inform the industry and agency staff on FDA thinking and expectations on certain subjects. Guidance documents do not create or confer any rights for or on any party or person and do not operate to bind FDA or the public.

There are two forms of guidance documents currently available from CDRH: the Blue Book Guidance Memoranda, which are older, informally issued guidances, and newer, formally issued guidance documents under the Good Guidance Practices regulation (GGP). The former are generally still available but will be replaced over time by the newer GGP guidances.

There are two types of GGP guidance documents:

- Level 1 guidances:

  - Set forth initial interpretations of statutory or regulatory requirements

  - Set forth changes in interpretation or policy that are of more than a minor nature

  - Include complex scientific issues

  - Cover highly controversial issues

- Level 2 guidances set forth existing practices or minor changes in interpretation or policy. Level 2 guidance documents include all guidance documents that are not classified as level 1.

Guidances may address general policy or procedural issues, deal with a specific scientific or clinical topic, or address issues related to a specific device type. If a manufacturer complies with the requirements of a guidance document, FDA is more likely to accept the actions of the manufacturer as consistent with FDA's expectations. However, if a manufacturer decides to take an approach that deviates from an applicable guidance, the burden of proof will be on the manufacturer to demonstrate that its approach is adequate and acceptable under the applicable legal or regulatory requirements. As in the use of consensus standards, FDA may obtain any information authorized by the applicable statute or regulations, including data substantiating conformance with a guidance document. Also, FDA may inspect and audit such information to confirm compliance with the identified guidance document.

CDRH guidance documents are available on the web and can be found at:

http://www.fda.gov/MedicalDevices/DeviceRegulationand Guidance/GuidanceDocuments/default.htm

FDA regulations, at 21 CFR 10.115(b)(3), provide examples of FDA documents that are not covered by GGP:

- Documents relating to internal FDA procedures

- Agency reports

- General information documents provided to consumers and health professionals

- Speeches

- Journal articles and editorials

- Media interviews and press materials

- Warning letters

- Other communications directed to individual persons or firms

PART 6. FDA ADMINISTRATIVE ACTIONS

FDA has the authority to undertake various administrative actions in administering the FDCA. These actions include: the promulgation of regulations that explain in further detail the requirements of the law; the conduct of various administrative hearings; holding advisory committee meetings; adoption of mandatory standards; issuing Warning Letters, Application Integrity Policy (AIP) letters, and deficiency letters; hearing and judging appeals; and acting on citizens' petitions.

FDA's compliance actions and enforcement of the law and regulations are discussed throughout the book in relation to specific topics and, in particular, appear in: Chapter 4, part 6, Bioresearch Monitoring; Chapter 7, part 13, QSIT Inspections; and Chapter 8, Compliance and Enforcement.

This part provides summary information on the promulgation of regulations, the conduct of hearings, and the adoption of mandatory standards.

Section 1. FDA Regulations

It is not the writing of the laws—it is their execution.

—Thomas Jefferson

The Importance of FDA Regulations

There are those who think that it is not necessary for professional practitioners in the medical device field to have a working knowledge of the regulations applicable to the design and development of a medical device and that their only responsibility is of a scientific and engineering nature. This could not be farther from the truth. The United States Food and Drug Administration will be there every step along the way once a device concept is adopted and work begins to develop a marketable medical device.

Due to the essential and critical role of engineers, other scientists, and health care practitioners in the development of a medical device, it is important for them to conduct their activities in a manner that meets the regulatory requirements that may be applicable. Failure to do so may result in serious penalties for either the individual practitioner or the manufacturer, or both.

The FDCA authorizes the Secretary of the Department of Health and Human Services to enforce the provisions of the act. The secretary, in turn, has delegated most of these authorities to the Commissioner of the Food and Drug Administration who has made further delegations related to medical devices to the Director of the Center for Devices and Radiological Health. Further delegations have been made, but for the purposes of this book, all administrative authorities and actions will be attributed to the FDA or CDRH, unless otherwise noted.

FDA's administration of the law includes many different types of actions. An important action of the FDA is the promulgation of rules and regulations. Its voluminous regulations are found in Title 21 of the Code of Federal Regulations, which can be found and searched on the FDA website at:

http://www.accessdata.fda.gov/scripts/cdrh/cfdocs/cfcfr/cfrsearch.cfm

These regulations have the full force and effect of law and they can be legally enforced by FDA through various administrative actions and judicial processes. FDA's regulations are so important that they constitute the main concentration of the materials in this book and their application to the design, testing, manufacture, and distribution of medical devices.

Promulgation of Regulations

In promulgating regulations, FDA must follow precise procedures as required by the Administrative Procedures Act and its own procedural requirements. The process of promulgating a regulation consists of three primary steps: publishing a proposed regulation, reviewing public comments, and publishing the final rule.

Proposing the Regulation

The first step in adopting a new or amended regulation is the publication of the proposal in the *Federal Register*, the official legal notification publication of the federal government. In addition to the publication of the proposal, a copy of the proposal is also included on the "public docket" and made available for anyone to read. Proposals are now also included on the Internet so interested parties do not have to travel to the agency's public docket office to read the proposal.

Sometimes the agency will publish what is known as an Advance Notice of Proposed Rulemaking, or ANPRM. This notice is used when the agency wants to let the public know what its preliminary thinking is and to allow the public to tender ideas on, support of, or objections to the agency's thinking.

A proposed regulation will be accompanied by a "preamble," which will describe in varying degrees of detail the intent and meaning of the proposed regulation. A draft of the proposed regulatory language will be included for review by the public. The proposal will also include a specified comment period during which time the public may submit comments. The proposal will include the name and contact information of a person who will manage the process for that regulation.

Accepting and Reviewing Public Comments

The second step in the regulatory process is the acceptance and review of comments received by FDA. In this context, any private individual, medical device manufacturer, institution, association, or public interest organization may submit comments on the proposed regulation. Comments may oppose the entire concept of the proposal, may oppose specific sections of the proposed regulation, may support any or all of the provisions, or may suggest additions, deletions, or amendments to the proposal.

All comments submitted to the agency will be reviewed and considered. The agency has to decide which comments to accept and which ones to reject.

Publishing the Final Regulation

After review and consideration of the comments received on the proposed regulation, the agency will prepare the final regulation. Sometimes, for very controversial proposals, the agency may choose to republish a modified proposal for a second round of comments. When the agency has made a final decision on the final language of the regulation, it will publish the final along with a preamble that will discuss all of the comments received, along with the agency's rationale for accepting or rejecting each comment. As needed, further explanation will be included to make the requirements of the regulation as clear as possible. The final regulation will include an effective date by which all affected parties must comply.

Section 2. Mandatory Standards

In addition to the recognition of voluntary consensus standards, FDA may adopt, through the promulgation of a regulation, mandatory standards applicable to a specific class of devices or to a specific device. Manufacturers must comply with mandatory standards if required by FDA. Many mandatory standards can be found in the classification regulations as discussed in this chapter, part 13, Medical Devices, Drugs, and Biologics.

Section 3. Administrative Hearings

Another major tool used by FDA in the administration of its responsibilities under the FDCA is the conduct of administrative hearings. In the broadest sense, any meeting with FDA may be considered an informal hearing. Such meetings would include pre-IDE (investigational device exemption) meetings, 510(k) and PMA meetings, informal appeals during the application review process, and other presentations to the agency that are not covered by a specific regulation related to the hearings.

There are essentially five types of generic hearings provided for in the regulations, which are identified by the part of Title 21 of the regulations under which they fall. In addition to these generic hearings, the regulations also provide for some exclusive subject matter hearings such as civil money penalties hearings under 21 CFR Part 17.

Part 12—Formal Evidentiary Public Hearing

A Part 12 hearing is used when a section of the FDCA specifically provides to a party the opportunity for such a hearing. These hearings are somewhat like a trial, with representation by attorneys, applicable rules of procedure, the presentation of evidence and witnesses, cross-examination, and an ultimate decision by an administrative law judge. An example of this type of hearing can be found in Section 515(g) of the FDCA, which provides for this type of hearing on an order approving or denying approval of a PMA application, as well as other agency actions.

Part 13—Hearing before a Public Board of Inquiry

A Part 13 hearing is applicable when (1) the regulations provide for a board hearing, (2) a party that is entitled to a Part 12 hearing waives that right and requests a Part 13 hearing, or (3) the commissioner determines that it is in the public interest to hold a public hearing before a board on any matter before FDA. These hearings are conducted as a scientific inquiry rather than a trial, and relevant scientific and technical data and information are presented to the board by participating parties.

Part 14—Hearing before a Public Advisory Committee

A Part 14 hearing is the type of hearing that will be encountered very frequently by medical device manufacturers, sponsors, and applicants because advisory committees play a significant role in providing scientific and medical advice to FDA and making recommendations to FDA on the approvability and conditions of use of new device applications. Medical device advisory committee review is discussed in detail in Chapter 5, part 1, Global Marketing Application Concepts.

Part 15—Public Hearing before the Commissioner

A Part 15 hearing may occur when (1) the FDCA or regulations provide for a hearing before the commissioner, (2) a party that is entitled to a Part 12 hearing waives that right and requests a Part 15 hearing, or (3) the commissioner determines that it is in the public interest to hold a public hearing on any matter before FDA. This type of hearing may be held, for example, to allow a party to propose device good manufacturing practice regulations. The commissioner does not always conduct these hearings personally, and frequently delegates this responsibility to others unless the regulation specifies that the commissioner must personally conduct this hearing.

Part 16—Regulatory Hearing before the Food and Drug Administration

A Part 16 hearing may be used any time the agency determines that additional information is desirable before taking a regulatory action. There are also many sections in the FDCA or regulations where the opportunity for this type of hearing is made available. The commissioner may appoint any qualified FDA employee as the presiding officer for this type of hearing.

PART 7. JUDICIAL REVIEW

Under the American legal system, the ultimate authority to interpret the meaning and intent of the law and to enforce it lies in the courts of the judicial branch of government. The courts have the constitutional responsibility to make the final decisions on the applicability of laws or regulations to particular situations and their enforcement by the government. Under their constitutional authority, the courts have the final say on whether FDA, in any particular case, has correctly interpreted and applied the law and regulations or whether the regulated party is in compliance with the law and regulations. The courts discharge their constitutional responsibilities through litigation, or court cases, in civil lawsuits, criminal prosecutions, and judicial review of agency actions.

Section 1. Agency Enforcement Actions

When FDA's administrative procedures are inadequate to deal with violative acts by a member of the regulated industry, FDA may turn to the courts, through various civil and criminal actions, to enforce the provisions of the act or regulations. These actions are discussed in Chapter 8, Compliance and Enforcement.

Section 2. Challenging Agency Actions

Just as FDA may turn to the courts for enforcement of the law, a regulated person may appeal to the courts for judicial review of an FDA action. A reviewing court may overturn or reverse an agency action if it finds any of the following to be true:

- The agency exceeded its statutory authority.

- The agency acted in an unreasonable or arbitrary manner.

- The agency failed to follow appropriate administrative procedures as required by the Administrative Procedures Act, the agency's own procedural requirements, or the established principles of administrative law.

- The law or regulation that was being enforced was unconstitutional.

PART 8. STATE REGULATION OF MEDICAL DEVICES

Section 1. Model Uniform State Food, Drug, and Cosmetic Act

Some states have their own medical device laws. State laws are generally local variations of the Model Uniform State Food, Drug, and Cosmetic Act. See for example, Connecticut Food, Drug, and Cosmetic Act, which can be found at:

> http://www.cga.ct.gov/2009/PUB/chap418.htm#Sec21a-91.htm

States also adopt regulations affecting medical devices. Both the laws and regulations follow the federal scheme of regulation of foods, drugs, and devices.

Section 2. Preemption of State Laws and Regulations

The FDCA expressly preempts any state law or regulation that is in derogation of federal requirements. Section 521 of the FDCA states:

(a) General rule

Except as provided in subsection (b) of this section, no State or political subdivision of a State may establish or continue in effect with respect to a device intended for human use any requirement—

1. which is different from, or in addition to, any requirement applicable under this chapter to the device, and

2. which relates to the safety or effectiveness of the device or to any other matter included in a requirement applicable to the device under this chapter.

Thus, state laws and regulations could supplement but not contradict the federal regulatory scheme. Congress felt that if a substantial number of differing requirements applicable to a medical device were imposed by jurisdictions other than the federal government, interstate commerce would be unduly burdened.

Under this preemption provision, if a state medical device requirement were challenged in court and it was found to be in derogation of the federal regulation of medical devices, the state provision would be found to be unenforceable.

It has been generally accepted that this preemption applies to statutory or regulatory requirements by a state. It is more contentious when there is an attempt to apply preemption to tort actions in a state court based on injuries sustained from the use of a medical device. This latter issue is very complex and beyond the scope of this book. The outcome of an affirmative preemption defense in a tort case may depend on whether the claim is against a 510(k) or PMA device, the exact requirements established by FDA, and other legal considerations.

PART 9. INTERNATIONAL ASPECTS OF DEVICE REGULATION

Many nations have some form of regulations for medical devices. The more developed nations have more sophisticated regulatory systems while the developing countries have relatively simplified systems. The laws and regulations of countries outside the United States are beyond the scope of this book because of the extent, variety, and complexity of those laws and regulations. This complexity is amply demonstrated by the following brief discussion of the medical device regulatory system in the European Union and the activities and efforts of the Global Harmonization Task Force.

It is worth noting that some countries that do not have an extensive regulatory system may request a copy of an FDA 510(k) letter or approval letter before allowing a company to import a medical device for commercial distribution. This practice has led some companies to seek FDA review of their products even though they intend to market the device outside of the United States.

Section 1. European Union Medical Device Regulation

The European Union (EU) is a supranational governmental organization consisting of 27 independent countries in Europe that have transferred some of their sovereignty or lawmaking authority to the EU. In the area of medical devices, each member country retains its authority to regulate medical devices within its border. However, the EU has the authority to harmonize these laws and has done so primarily through the issuance of "directives," which are harmonizing standards.

EU Legal Framework

Directives require member states to achieve a certain result while leaving them discretion as to how to achieve the result. The details of how they are to be implemented are left to member states. Directives normally leave member states with a certain amount of leeway as to the exact rules to be adopted. At the present time there are three major directives affecting medical devices:

- Medical Devices—Council Directive 93/42/EEC

- Active Implantable Medical Devices—Council Directive 90/385/EEC of 20 June 1990

- In Vitro Diagnostic Medical Devices—Directive 98/79/EC

According to the *Report on the Issue of the Reprocessing of Medical Devices in the European Union, in Accordance with Article 12a of Directive 93/42/EEC:*

> These three legal texts form the core legal framework for medical devices. Their aim is both to ensure a high level of protection of human health and safety and the functioning of the internal market.

The requirements of these directives are incorporated into the national laws of member states, who may add to but not subtract from directives. For those readers seeking more information on the EU medical device regulatory system, a good starting place is the European Union Consumer Affairs website at:

http://ec.europa.eu/consumers/sectors/medical-devices/index_en.htm

Marketing a Medical Device in the EU

In order for a manufacturer to commercially distribute a medical device within the European market, the requirements of the EU directives have to be met. Manufacturers' products meeting these harmonized standards have a presumption of conformity to the directive. Products conforming with the Medical Device (MD) Directive must have a CE mark applied, which indicates conformity.

A CE mark is obtained from a "Notified Body," which is responsible for verifying conformance to the law. There is at least one Notified Body per EU member, and there are more than 27 Notified Bodies in all. A Notified Body of particular interest to the United States medical device industry is G-MED North America, a subsidiary of LNE/G-MED, a French Notified Body for the European directives covering medical devices. G-MED NA is located in the Washington, D.C., area and offers:

> . . . a comprehensive range of solutions for medical device manufacturers and their subcontractors in North America:
>
> - Product assessment for CE marking: in accordance with the European Directives on medical devices
>
> - Certification of company management systems
>
> - Quality certification of sterilization processes
>
> - Certification for access to the Canadian and American markets
>
> - Specific training on request

LNE/G-MED's notification covers all categories of medical devices and all assessment procedures, including the type of approval, the approval of quality management systems, and EC verification.

Further:

> For the medical device Directives 90/385/EEC, 93/42/EC, 98/79/EC, 2000/70/EC and 2003/32/EC, LNE/G-MED will:
>
> - Provide information on regulations and certification procedures
>
> - Provide an expert opinion concerning classification of devices
>
> - Issue the certificates required for CE marking
>
> - Carry out EC examinations of design files
>
> - Carry out EC type examinations
>
> - Carry out EC verifications
>
> - Perform conformity tests to harmonized European standards or other standards
>
> - Perform quality system audits in accordance with the annexes of the Directives

- Assess clinical, biological, or scientific data, in consultation with hospital experts when required

The LNE/G-MED website contains extensive information on the requirements applicable to medical devices in the EU and can be found at:

http://www.lne-gmed.com/en/services/ce-marking.asp

Section 2. Global Harmonization Task Force

Just as the EU has maintained a process for harmonizing the medical device requirements within its member states, there is a parallel international effort to bring some consistency and uniformity to the laws and regulations of the various countries and jurisdictions with medical device laws and regulations. This effort is spearheaded by the Global Harmonization Task Force (GHTF), which was founded by the United States, Canada, the European Union, Australia, and Japan. FDA is very active in the efforts of the GHTF. According to FDA:

> The GHTF fosters international harmonization in the regulation of medical devices. Regulatory and industry authorities from Europe, Asia-Pacific, and North America collaborate to encourage the harmonization of regulatory practices to ensure the safety, effectiveness, and quality of medical devices.

As described on its website, the GHTF:

> . . . was conceived in 1992 in an effort to achieve greater uniformity between national medical device regulatory systems. This is being done with two aims in mind: enhancing patient safety and increasing access to safe, effective, and clinically beneficial medical technologies around the world.
>
> A partnership between regulatory authorities and regulated industry, the GHTF is comprised of five Founding Members: European Union, United States, Canada, Australia, and Japan. The chairmanship is rotated among the Founding Members and presently resides with Australia.
>
> Currently GHTF has five Study Groups that address premarket through post-market medical device issues.

- Study Group 1—Premarket Evaluation

- Study Group 2—Post-Market Surveillance/ Vigilance

- Study Group 3—Quality Systems

- Study Group 4—Auditing

- Study Group 5—Clinical Safety/Performance

These study groups study inconsistencies and conflicts between international requirements, provide findings, and make recommendations to the international community on changes that might be made in national laws, regulations, and policies that will tend to normalize the various regulatory requirements among countries. One result of these efforts is demonstrated in the discussion of ISO Voluntary Audit Reports in Chapter 7, part 13, section 3, Third-Party Inspections. Another effect is the recognition by FDA of inspections conducted by other member states when determining the inspection it will conduct under U.S. law.

The GHTF maintains its website at:

http://www.ghtf.org/

Section 3. Other Requirements with International Implications

There are certain requirements within the U.S. regulatory system for medical devices that relate to international commerce in medical devices or that have a direct bearing on the marketing of a medical device in the United States. For example, gathering test data outside of the United States is discussed in Chapter 4, part 1, section 2, International Guidelines for Medical Device Research; the import and export of investigational medical devices is covered in Chapter 4, part 7, Importing and Exporting Medical Devices for Investigational Use; the use of foreign research data in marketing applications is dealt with in Chapter 5, part 1, section 2, Valid Scientific Evidence; the import or export of medical devices for marketing purposes is discussed in Chapter 5, part 4, Importing and Exporting Medical Devices for Commercial Distribution; and the application of consensus standards developed by international organizations is presented above in part 5, Quasi-Legal Requirements.

PART 10. CONFIDENTIALITY AND NONPUBLIC INFORMATION

A topic of importance to both industry and FDA employees is the confidentiality of information with which they deal. This topic is universal and is not confined to the topics discussed in any one chapter of this book. Therefore, it is discussed here because it can apply to many of the topics discussed throughout this book.

Section 1. Nonpublic Information

There are several types of data and information that fall under the rubric of nondisclosable or nonpublic information. The major ones of interest in this book are: trade secrets, confidential commercial information, financially sensitive information, personal patient information, and personal employee information. It is safe to say that all medical device companies possess some protected data, and many companies possess a great deal of data and information that are considered to be privileged.

The types of data and information discussed in the following sections are considered to be nonpublic and, therefore, subject to protection under company confidentiality agreements or under laws and regulations applicable to FDA employees.

Section 2. Trade Secrets

Trade secret information consists of secret formulae, schematics, materials, and processes without which the product could not be duplicated. The classic and well-known example of a trade secret is the carefully guarded formula for making Coca-Cola syrup.

Because of the importance of trade secret information in business and commerce, there has been a long tradition in Anglo-American law protecting a person's trade secret information. In order for information to fall under the protection of law as a trade secret, it must, in the first instance, be a secret. If a company does not treat the information in a protected manner or publishes, or lets be published, the information, then the information would no longer be considered a "trade secret." Any information that would otherwise be considered a trade secret that makes its way into the "public domain," from whatever legal source, would not qualify as a secret and, therefore, not be subject to protection as a trade secret.

Companies treat trade secrets so seriously that many companies will honor the trade secret status of a competitor's information. Several years ago, a highly placed employee of the Coca-Cola Company offered to sell the Coke formula to an executive of PepsiCo Inc. PepsiCo reported this to the Coca-Cola Company and the Coca-Cola employee was discharged by her employer for violation of the confidentiality agreement under which she was bound.

FDA receives a great deal of trade secret information in submissions from manufacturers. The FDCA has a special provision for the treatment of trade secrets received by the FDA. It provides, in Section 520(c):

> Trade secrets. Any information reported to or otherwise obtained by the Secretary or his representative under section 513, 514, 515, 516, 518, 519, or 704 or under subsection (f) or (g) of this section which is exempt from disclosure pursuant to subsection (a) of section 552 of title 5, United States Code, by reason of subsection (b)(4) of such section shall be considered confidential and shall not be disclosed and may not be used by the Secretary as the basis for the reclassification of a device from class III to class II or class I or as the basis for the establishment or amendment of a performance standard under section 514 for a device reclassified from class III to class II, except (1) in accordance with subsection (h), and (2) that such information may be disclosed to other officers or employees concerned with carrying out this Act or when relevant in any proceeding under this Act (other than section 513 or 514 thereof).

The referenced Section 552 of Title 5 of the United States Code, subsection (b)(4), exempts from disclosure under the Freedom of Information Act (FOIA):

> (4) trade secrets and commercial or financial information obtained from a person and privileged or confidential

The FDCA also makes it a crime for an FDA employee to disclose trade secret information outside of the DHHS. Section 303(a)(1), Penalties, states:

> Any person who violates a provision of section 301 shall be imprisoned for not more than one year or fined not more than $1,000, or both.

Section 301, Prohibited Acts, states, in part:

> The following acts and the causing thereof are hereby prohibited:
>
> ...
>
> (j) The using by any person to his own advantage or revealing, other than to the Secretary or officers or employees of the Department, or to the courts when relevant in any judicial proceeding under this Act, any information acquired under authority of section 404, 409, 412, 414, 505, 510, 512, 513, 514, 515, 516, 518, 519, 520, 571, 572, 573, 704, 708, or 721 concerning any method

or process which as a trade secret is entitled to protection; or the violating of section 408(i)(2) or any regulation issued under that section. This paragraph does not authorize the withholding of information from either House of Congress or from, to the extent of matter within its jurisdiction, any committee or subcommittee of such committee or any joint committee of Congress or any subcommittee of such joint committee.

Hence, the release or disclosure of trade secret information by an FDA employee is subject to criminal penalties under the law.

Section 3. Confidential Commercial Information

Confidential commercial information (CCI) is less clearly defined than trade secret information because it depends on the importance of the information in the conduct of the company's business. At a minimum, the information must be kept confidential by the company and be of a nature such that if released and known to competitors, it could harm or impair the owner's competitive advantage in having that information.

The types of information considered to be CCI are generally of a business nature rather than technical or scientific. This would include records such as sources of supply, production and marketing costs, customer lists, and employee information.

As stated above, the FOIA includes commercial or financial information in the exemption from disclosure.

Section 4. Financially Sensitive Information

Financially sensitive company information may consist of cost data related to supplies or services, manufacturing or marketing costs, pricing information or profit margins, or other expenditures related to the development, testing, or distribution of a medical device. Knowing a company's financial information could help a competitor gain an advantage in competing with the company.

Other financially sensitive information may relate to the status of a company's marketing applications. This type of information is frequently sought by some financial advisors and investors who may be in a position to make substantial sums of money in the stock market if they can obtain insider information concerning the approval or disapproval of a pending application under review by FDA.

Section 5. Specific Patient Information

Patient information is protected under law and regulation as a right to privacy. Section 552(b) of the FOIA exempts in subsection (6):

> (6) personnel and medical files and similar files the disclosure of which would constitute a clearly unwarranted invasion of personal privacy

Thus, federal agencies, including FDA, do not have to release this type of information under the FOIA.

Health Insurance Portability and Accountability Act of 1996 (HIPAA)

Other federal laws, such as the Health Insurance Portability and Accountability Act of 1996 (HIPAA) and its regulations, control the protection and disclosure of patient information. HIPAA requirements are extremely important to those in the private sector or within government agencies who, as part of their professional practice or in their conduct of the clinical testing of a medical device, acquire personal health data from patients or subjects. The HIPAA Privacy Rule includes all "providers of services" (for example, institutional providers such as hospitals) and "providers of medical or health services" (for example, noninstitutional providers such as physicians, dentists, and other practitioners) as defined by Medicare, and any other person or organization that furnishes, bills, or is paid for healthcare. For those interested, additional information about HIPAA can be found on the DHHS website at:

> http://www.hhs.gov/ocr/privacy/index.html

Whether a party sponsoring or conducting research of a medical device is covered by the HIPAA rules depends on many factors. As a general rule, research itself is not covered by HIPAA. However, the institutions where the research is conducted and those institutions or providers of services providing the data and information on which the research is based are most likely covered by the HIPAA rules. Extensive guidance on how the HIPAA Privacy Rule applies to research can be found on the DHHS website at:

> http://www.hhs.gov/ocr/privacy/hipaa/understanding/
> coveredentities/research.html

Whether or not HIPAA rules apply to any particular research on a medical device, it is important to understand that FDA rules will, nevertheless, be applicable and must be followed. These FDA rules are discussed in detail in Chapter 4, Clinical Trials.

Section 6. Specific Employee Information

Just as patients do not want their personal information released without their permission, neither do employees of a company or FDA employees want their personal information released to individuals who are not connected with their employer. The purpose of such records is for the employment and business purposes of the employer, and as such this type of information is considered nondisclosable and protected zealously by employers. As with other protected information provided to FDA, the agency does not have to release this type of information under the FOIA, as stated in the quote from Section 552(b)(6), above.

Section 7. Protecting Nonpublic Information

To prevent the unauthorized release of privileged information in the private sector, a company employee is generally bound by a *confidentiality agreement*, which prohibits the employee from disclosing nonpublic information in the files of the company. This information, however, may be shared by the company with its outside contractors and agents for business purposes. In such cases, there generally would be a confidentiality agreement between the parties to protect the business and commercial interests of both parties.

A company will frequently submit or be asked to submit, or may be required by law or regulation to submit, privileged data and information in submissions made to FDA for review and evaluation. This occurs most frequently during the review of premarket evaluation submissions, but it can also occur in submissions related to compliance matters and post-market reports.

FDA employees, however, are not bound by confidentiality agreements with the submitting companies as their private sector counterparts are. Rather, agency employees sign nondisclosure agreements with FDA and are prohibited by law and regulation from disclosing nonpublic information. As pointed out above, an FDA employee, under Section 301(j), may not disclose manufacturing methods or processes that constitute trade secret information submitted to the agency to anyone who is not an employee of the DHHS.

As a result of the foregoing restrictions on the disclosure of nonpublic information, agency employees are very careful not to disclose protected information received from the regulated industry. As an added protection, agency employees will discuss a company's pending business before the agency only with the person designated by the company as the *official correspondent*. The official correspondent may be an employee of the company, an outside consultant, or the company's legal counsel, as specified by the company.

There are, however, certain conditions under which the agency may share nonpublic information with parties who are not DHHS employees. These exceptions do not contravene statutory restrictions because of the manner in which they are implemented. For example, the agency may share nonpublic information with its contractors, who must sign nondisclosure agreements and who are subject to the same legal and regulatory restrictions as an FDA employee. Another example would be where the agency shares 301(j) protected information with a foreign government agent who is visiting FDA for training purposes or for the purpose of conducting a joint review, if the submitter of the protected information authorizes such disclosure in writing.

The primary types of protection for nonpublic information in the private and public sectors are demonstrated in Figure 1.4.

PART 11. MONITORING AND AUDITING

Both monitoring and auditing are processes that constitute a review of actions that have taken place in regard to the design, testing, or manufacturing of a medical device.

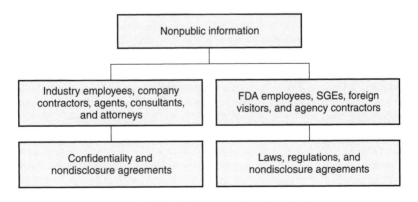

Figure 1.4   Protection of nonpublic information.

Section 1. Monitoring

Monitoring is a less intensive process than auditing. A monitor typically will examine the records related to a process to make sure all of the necessary steps have been executed, without necessarily examining the substance of the records to assure accuracy and verifiability. If a monitor observes incorrect information in a record during the monitoring process, the appropriate correction most likely will be made, but that is not the primary purpose of the activity. The primary purpose of the monitoring is to verify the process itself.

Clinical Trial Monitoring

For example, the monitor of a clinical trial will review the clinical trial records to determine whether the clinical investigator and the clinical trial staff have obtained signed informed consent forms from the study subjects, whether the necessary communications have taken place with the institutional review board (IRB), whether the case report forms have been completed, and whether other requirements for conducting a clinical trial have been met. The monitor will not necessarily determine whether the data entered in the case report forms (CRFs) are accurate and complete.

On the other hand, an auditor will be examining the same clinical trial records in order to verify the accuracy and completeness of the data and information in the records. For the same clinical trial, for example, a complete and thorough audit will compare the data in each subject's medical record to the data entered on the CRF. The data on the CRF will then be compared to the data that were used for, or submitted in, an application to the FDA. Any discrepancies or omissions that are discovered would have to be corrected so the final database on which the submission is based is accurate, complete, and reliable.

Section 2. Auditing

Auditing is an intensive and expensive process and is at times either necessary or required. It can be used for a variety of purposes.

Due Diligence Audit When Purchasing a Company or a Product

Auditing can be used when one company is purchasing another company. For example, if company A is purchasing company B, the general rule is that A will conduct a "due diligence" audit of B to be sure they are getting what they bargained for. In doing so, the auditor for A will audit the business records of B to confirm the financial status of B, the product lines, the personnel, the regulatory status of B and its products, and so on.

Auditing may also be used in the purchase of a product. For example, if company A is purchasing a medical device from company B, or the marketing license to the device for the purpose of obtaining a new product that has been clinically tested by B, A may want to conduct a full audit of the data generated by A's clinical trial to be sure they are complete and accurate so they may be submitted to FDA. There have been cases in which the purchasing company used—without auditing—the data and information generated by the purchased company as the basis for a submission to FDA only to find out that the data were unreliable and, therefore, false or misleading in the eyes of the agency. This has resulted in an Application Integrity Policy (AIP) action against the purchasing company to the detriment of the company's fortunes and reputation.

AIP Data and System Audit

Companies under an AIP action are required by FDA to conduct a complete pass-through audit of the data starting with the medical record and proceeding to the CRFs and the FDA submission as described immediately above. Without this complete audit, and other requirements, the AIP will stay in effect, and applications will not be accepted and reviewed by the agency. This, in effect, will prohibit the company from marketing new devices. Even when an AIP action is removed, the company may be required to include such data audits on all new applications for a certain period of time, usually two years.

AIP audits also include a company- or firm-wide system audit. The purpose of this audit is to determine what systemwide deficiencies, for example, inadequately trained personnel or lack of appropriate standard operating procedures (SOPs), led to the collection, storage, analysis, and submission of false or misleading statements.

The AIP program and its requirements are discussed in Chapter 5, part 1, section 7, Data Integrity.

QSR Auditing

Auditing is also required under the Quality System Regulation (QSR) when problems arise with a marketed device. For example, when a medical device is recalled, the recalling manufacturer may, depending on the problem underlying the recall, conduct an audit of the design, testing, or manufacturing of the device to determine the underlying cause of the problem. Such an audit may be necessary in order to establish an acceptable CAPA under QSR. Discussions of quality audits and CAPA audits appear in Chapter 7, part 1, Management and Organization, and part 8, Corrective and Preventive Actions.

PART 12. PATENTS

The purpose of the patent system is to promote the exchange of information about scientific discoveries and inventions. Patents may contain formulae, schematics, processes, and so on, that are in the nature of trade secret information. However, under patent law, the content of a patent is made available to any member of the public. Inventors, in exchange for public disclosure, are granted 18 years of exclusive use.

Patent Restoration

A problem arose under the patent system in relation to FDA-regulated products. An inventor, such as a medical device or drug manufacturer, would file a patent as soon as possible to protect the rights to its invention. The clock on the 18 years of patent protection would then begin to run. The time it took the inventor to complete the required FDA testing, studies, and premarket review might consume years of the patent protection period. To restore the intended benefits of the patent protection time period to products regulated by FDA, in 1984 Congress enacted the Drug Price Competition and Patent Term Restoration Act to add time to the patent period for time lost due to the FDA clearance process.

PART 13. MEDICAL DEVICES, DRUGS, AND BIOLOGICS

FDA regulates several types of products intended for the treatment of humans. It is important to distinguish between medical devices and the other closely related products that fall within FDA's regulatory sphere. Sometimes these products are used in combination. This part considers the differences between devices, drugs, and biological products and describes the types and classification of devices. Furthermore, the classification of a device is critically important because it will determine which regulatory requirements have to be met.

Section 1. Medical Devices

Medical devices, as regulated by FDA, are defined in Section 201(h) of the FDCA, which states:

(h) The term "device" . . . means an instrument, apparatus, implement, machine, contrivance, implant, in vitro reagent, or other similar or related article, including any component, part, or accessory, which is—

(1) recognized in the official National Formulary, or the United States Pharmacopeia, or any supplement to them,

(2) intended for use in the diagnosis of disease or other conditions, or in the cure, mitigation, treatment, or prevention of disease, in man or other animals, or

(3) intended to affect the structure or any function of the body of man or other animals, and which does not achieve its primary intended purposes through chemical action within or on the body of man or other animals *and which is not dependent upon being metabolized for the achievement of its primary intended purposes.* (Emphasis Added.)

This definition recognizes that medical devices are composed of mechanical parts, electrical circuitry, computer-controlled functions, new and exotic materials, communication functions, and, actually, any materials or components of devices and equipment in general. There are approximately 1700 generic types of devices.

General Medical Devices

- General purpose reagent

- Electrocardiograph

- Latex patient examination gloves

- Piston syringe

- Endoscope

- Dental floss

- Replacement heart valve

- Combination products consisting of a device and a therapeutic drug, controlled substance, or biological product

In Vitro Diagnostic Devices

In vitro diagnostic devices (IVDs) are tests that can detect diseases, conditions, or infections. As such, they fall within the definition of a medical device. Some tests are used in laboratory or other health professional settings, and other tests are for consumers to use at home. The bulk of medical device requirements, as covered in this book, apply to IVDs, with several exceptions, primarily in the area of evaluation. Further information about IVD regulatory requirements can be found on the IVD home page at:

http://www.fda.gov/MedicalDevices/DeviceRegulationand
Guidance/IVDRegulatoryAssistance/default.htm

Radiation Emitting Devices

Radiation emitting devices intended for medical use may be used for diagnostic, therapeutic, and surgical purposes and for other medical applications. These devices are regulated as medical devices and subject to the same requirements as other medical devices. Radiation emitting medical devices are also subject to the requirements of the Radiation Control for Health and Safety Act of 1968 (RCHSA), which has been incorporated into the FDCA. Radiation emitting medical devices are, therefore, regulated by FDA under the authority of both the FDCA and the RCHSA. It may also be noted that some of these medical devices are further subject to the requirements of the Mammography Quality Standards Act of 1992.

Other radiation emitting devices not intended for medical use, such as those with scientific, industrial, business, commercial, and security uses, are also regulated by FDA under the RCHSA. Under the RCHSA and its regulations, all radiation emitting devices, whether for medical use or not, must meet a variety of requirements that are beyond the scope of this book. Anyone wishing to explore the world of radiation emitting devices and their regulation by FDA may consult the following website:

http://www.fda.gov/Radiation-EmittingProducts/default.htm

Combination Products and Medical Device Jurisdiction

Within FDA, the Center for Devices and Radiological Health (CDRH) has primary responsibility for the regulation of medical devices. However, some medical devices combined with drugs or biologics may be regulated jointly with, or primarily by, the Center for Drug Evaluation and Research (CDER) or the Center for Biologics Evaluation and Research (CBER). These products are discussed in section 8, Combination Products, below.

Section 2. Drug Products

The italicized language in the statutory definition above distinguishes a medical device from a drug under this law. Hence, a drug is a product that utilizes *chemical action* and *is metabolized* to achieve its intended purpose in the treatment or diagnosis of a disease or condition in a human being. Examples of drug products include:

- Analgesics

- Antibiotics

- Antidepressants

- Hormone replacement therapies

- Anti-inflammatory agents

- Growth steroids

- Cholinergic and anticholinergic drugs

- Cold and cough preparations

- Anesthetics

Within FDA, CDER has primary responsibility for the regulation of drug products.

Section 3. Biological Products

It is also important to distinguish a regulated biological product from a medical device. Biologics are subject to regulation under the FDCA because most biological products also meet the definition of drugs or devices as defined in the act. However, it should be noted that biologics are also subject to regulation under Section 262 of the Public Health Service Act (PHSA), which, among other requirements, provides for the licensing of biological products by the FDA before they may be introduced and distributed in interstate commerce. Furthermore, nothing contained in the biologics provisions of the PHSA may be construed as in any way affecting, modifying, repealing, or superseding the provisions of the FDCA.

Like medical devices and drugs, biological products are intended for use in prevention, treatment, or cure of diseases or injuries of man. Biological products replicate natural substances such as enzymes, antibodies, or hormones in our bodies. Biologics can be composed of sugars, proteins, or nucleic acids, or a combination of these substances. They may also be living entities, such as cells and tissue. Biologics are made from a variety of natural resources—human, animal, and microorganism—and may be produced by biotechnology methods. Examples of types of biologics include:

- Allergenic extracts (for example, for allergy shots and tests)

- Blood and blood components

- Gene therapy products

- Human tissue and cellular products used in transplantation

- Vaccines

- Monoclonal antibodies designed as targeted therapies in cancer and other diseases

- Cytokines (types of proteins involved in immune response)

- Growth factors (proteins that affect the growth of a cell)

- Enzymes (types of proteins that speed up biochemical reactions) such as thrombolytics (used to dissolve blood clots)

- Immunomodulators (agents that affect immune response)

Within FDA, CBER has primary responsibility for the regulation of biological products and some medical devices used to produce biologics.

Section 4. Classification of Medical Devices

The Medical Device Amendments of 1976 (MDA) directed FDA to classify all devices. There are about 1700 generic types of medical devices, which have been classified into three major classes of medical devices: Class I, Class II, and Class III. This is a risk-based classification system depending on the level of control necessary to assure the safety and effectiveness of the device. Each class is discussed separately below. See also the FDA device classification web page at:

> http://www.fda.gov/MedicalDevices/DeviceRegulationand
> Guidance/Overview/ClassifyYourDevice/default.htm

Classification Regulations

The FDCA includes various procedures for the classification of medical devices. Initially, devices were classified through the use of expert advisory panels that made classification recommendations. After comments from the general public were considered, FDA adopted final classification regulations that consisted of 16 categories or "panels" of medical devices based on the medical use of the device as identified in Table 1.2. Each classified device is identified under its own classification provision within the appropriate panel with its classification name and any special conditions or restrictions that apply to it.

Table 1.2 Classification panels for medical devices.

21 CFR Part	Medical specialty panel
862	Clinical chemistry and clinical toxicology devices
864	Hematology and pathology devices
866	Immunology and microbiology devices
868	Anesthesiology devices
870	Cardiovascular devices
872	Dental devices
874	Ear, nose, and throat devices
876	Gastroenterology and urology devices
878	General and plastic surgery devices
880	General hospital and personal use devices
882	Neurology devices
884	Obstetrical and gynecological devices
886	Ophthalmic devices
888	Orthopedic devices
890	Physical medicine devices
892	Radiology devices

Product Codes

In addition to being classified, each device is given a product code consisting of three letters. The product code can be used to search for a predicate device, to search Medical Device Reports (MDRs) in the public database, and to search listings in the public database. It is also used by FDA in planning its inspection assignments. Product codes can be found on all 510(k)/ PMA clearance/approval letters or in FDA's searchable Product Code Classification Database at:

> http://www.fda.gov/MedicalDevices/DeviceRegulationand
> Guidance/Overview/ClassifyYourDevice/ucm051637.htm

Reclassification

Since the enactment of MDA, all new devices have been classified automatically into Class III unless they were found to be substantially equivalent to a device in Class I or Class II. At any time after classification, and based on increased experience and knowledge about a device, FDA may, on its own or in response to an outside petition, change a device's classification by regulation. A manufacturer who wishes to have a device reclassified to a lower class must convince FDA that the less-stringent class requirements will be sufficient to provide reasonable assurance of safety and effectiveness.

Section 5. Classes of Medical Devices

Class I Devices—General Controls

Class I devices are the lowest-risk devices, for which "general controls," with or without exemptions, are sufficient to provide reasonable assurance of their safety and effectiveness because they are relatively low-risk devices. The safety and effectiveness of these devices is well known and the technology is well understood.

The term *general controls* refers to a wide range of responsibilities and requirements that are applicable to all manufacturers and others who are engaged in the medical device distribution system. *All devices, regardless of classification, must be in compliance with the general controls unless exempt.* These controls are discussed in Chapter 8, part 1, General Controls.

Class II Devices—Performance Standards

Devices are put into Class II, performance standards, if general controls are not sufficient to provide reasonable assurance of safety and effectiveness and there is sufficient information to establish a performance standard to provide reasonable assurance of safety and effectiveness. Class II devices are more complex and present a moderate risk when compared to Class I or Class III devices.

Class II devices must meet the "general control" provisions of the FDCA and, in addition, they must meet applicable "performance standards" developed by the FDA or by other governmental or private organizations whose offers to develop standards are accepted. The FDA also may adopt, by regulation, an existing standard. Standards are discussed above in Part 5, Quasi-Legal Requirements.

In addition to a mandatory performance standard, a specific Class II device may further be required to meet any special control established by FDA for that device or class of devices. The types of "special controls" that may be applicable include: the conduct of a post-market surveillance study, the establishment of patient registries, meeting a specific guideline, following agency recommendations or other actions, and using special labeling required for the device.

Class III Devices

Class III devices represent the highest-risk devices. They are designed for use in supporting or sustaining human health, or present a potential unreasonable risk of illness or injury, and there is insufficient information to establish a performance standard to assure their safety and effectiveness. In addition, Class III devices must be in compliance with the "general controls" and meet any "special controls" that may be applicable.

Class III devices are (1) pre-amendment devices that have been classified into Class III, (2) post-amendment devices that are not substantially equivalent to a pre-amendment device, or (3) transitional devices. Transitional devices are pre-amendment devices that have been approved under a new drug application for which FDA has not called for a PMA.

Premarket Approval

Class III products require FDA approval of a premarketing application. This approval process is discussed in detail in Chapter 5, Marketing Applications. These submissions are based on valid scientific evidence, such as well-controlled studies, that provide a reasonable assurance of the device's safety and effectiveness for human use.

Conditions of Approval

Class III devices are further subject to any conditions set forth in the approval order. These conditions may relate to the device's manufacture, packaging, labeling, distribution, use, or follow-up studies, and are discussed in Chapter 5, Marketing Applications.

Section 6. Class I and Class II Device Exemptions

Exemptions from certain regulatory requirements may apply to either Class I or Class II devices. To avoid the need to repeat this information under the discussions above for each of these device classes, the subject of exemptions is included here and applicable to the discussion of either class of devices as noted.

Premarket Notification (510[k]) Exemption

Most Class I devices and a few Class II devices are exempt from the 510(k) requirements, subject to the limitations on exemptions. Devices exempt from 510(k) are pre-amendment devices not significantly changed or modified, or Class I/II devices specifically exempted by regulation. If a manufacturer's device falls into a generic category of exempted Class I devices, a premarket notification application and FDA clearance are not required before marketing the device in the United States.

At the present time, FDA has exempted over 800 generic types of Class I devices and about 60 Class II devices from the premarket notification requirement. However, some devices that might otherwise be exempt from 510(k) have been designated "Reserved Medical Devices." See links immediately below.

General Controls Exemption

Devices exempt from 510(k) are not exempt from other general controls. For example, all medical devices must be manufactured under a quality assurance program, be suitable for the intended use, be adequately packaged and properly labeled, and have establishment registration and device listing forms on file with the FDA.

Good Manufacturing Practices (GMPs) Exemption

A few Class I devices that are exempt from the need to obtain 510(k) clearance are additionally exempt from the GMP requirements, with the exception of complaint files and general record-keeping requirements.

FDA Exemption Databases

The topic of exemptions can be confusing. The 510(k) exemption has certain limitations, so it is important to confirm the exempt status and any limitations that may apply to a specific device. These limitations, if any, are set forth in each device's classification regulation. These can be found in FDA's searchable Product Code Classification Database, as cited above, or in subsequent *Federal Register* announcements on Class I exemptions and Class II exemptions.

To avoid misunderstandings, FDA has placed on its website two pages that identify the devices that are exempt from 510(k) requirements and those exempt from both 510(k) and GMP requirements. Even within this comprehensive listing, it is important to pay attention to the footnotes for clarification. These pages are:

510(k) and GMP exemptions:

> http://www.accessdata.fda.gov/scripts/cdrh/cfdocs/
> cfpcd/315.cfm

Reserved Medical Devices:

> http://www.accessdata.fda.gov/scripts/cdrh/cfdocs/
> cfpcd/3151.cfm

Section 7. Restricted and Prescription Devices

The FDA is authorized to restrict the sale, distribution, or use of a device if its safety and effectiveness can not be reasonably assured through labeled instructions for use. These *restricted devices* are analogous to prescription drugs and must bear a similar legend.

As with prescription drugs, such devices may be dispensed or sold pursuant to the order of an individual authorized by state law to administer or prescribe such products. They are sold by pharmacists or other health professionals, for example, medical and surgical supply dealers authorized or otherwise permitted by state law to do so.

Section 8. Combination Products

There are three primary types of FDA-regulated products that may be used together in different forms such as: a drug and device, a device plus biologic, a drug and biologic, and a drug–device–biologic. These products are referred to as *combination products* and may be used for therapeutic or diagnostic purposes.

There are several ways in which the adjunctive use of these products becomes a combination product. It may be a product comprising two or more regulated components that are physically linked, two or more separate products packaged together, or two or more products packaged separately but required to be used together.

Some examples of combination medical device products include:

- Drug-eluting stents, antimicrobial or heparin-coated catheters, condoms with spermicidal coating, pacing leads with steroid-coated tips

- Skin substitutes with cellular components, orthopedic implants with growth factors, biologically based sealants, glues, and homeostatic agents

- Insulin/epinephrine/interferon injector pens, metered dose inhalers, transdermal patches

- Combinations of device components

Office of Combination Products

Because combination products involve components that would normally be regulated under different types of regulatory authorities, and frequently by different FDA Centers, they raise challenging regulatory, policy, and review challenges. Differences in regulatory pathways for each component can impact the regulatory processes for all aspects of product development and management, including preclinical testing, clinical investigation, marketing applications, manufacturing and quality control, adverse event reporting, promotion and advertising, and post-approval modifications.

To handle these potential conflicts in jurisdiction within FDA, the agency created the Office of Combination Products (OCP) at the agency level. The OCP assigns primary review responsibility for combination products to an appropriate Center within FDA. This assignment is based on the "primary mode of action" of the product.

Request for Designation

To start the process, a company will submit a "Request for Designation" to the OCP where a determination will be made concerning the primary mode of action after consultation with the appropriate Centers. Based on this determination, the product will be assigned to one Center as the lead for the review of the premarket application and regulation. During the review of the premarket application, the Centers will confer and consult with each other so that the review, evaluation, and regulation of the product reflect the combined evaluation of the appropriate Centers.

The Designation Rationale

An example of a combination product with device and drug components is the Gem 21S dental bone graft with growth factor. The primary purpose of this product is the repair of periodontal defects. The secondary action is for the drug component to promote growth of new bone. Since the primary mode of action is derived from the device component, the product is regulated by the CDRH as a device, and it would be reviewed through a PMA application.

Another example with a different outcome would be the Daytrana transdermal patch. The primary purpose of the patch is for the treatment of ADHD while the patch itself is merely a delivery system for the drug. Therefore this product is regulated by CDER as a drug under a New Drug Application (NDA).

Section 9. Custom Devices

A *custom device* is a device that is not generally available in finished form for purchase and is not offered through labeling or advertising by the manufacturer. The FDCA, Section 520(b), defines custom device in the following manner:

(b) Custom devices. Sections 514 and 515 do not apply to any device which, in order to comply with the order of an individual physician or dentist (or any other specially qualified person designated under regulations promulgated by the Secretary after an opportunity for an oral hearing) necessarily deviates from an otherwise applicable performance standard or requirement prescribed by or under section 515 if

(1) the device is not generally available in finished form for purchase or for dispensing upon prescription and is not offered through labeling or advertising by the manufacturer, importer, or distributor thereof for commercial distribution, and

(2) such device

(A)(i) is intended for use by an individual patient named in such order of such physician or dentist (or other specially qualified person so designated) and is to be made in a specific form for such patient, or

(ii) is intended to meet the special needs of such physician or dentist (or other specially qualified person so designated) in the course of the professional practice of such physician or dentist (or other specially qualified person so designated), and

(B) is not generally available to or generally used by other physicians or dentists (or other specially qualified persons so designated).

FDA provided a look at its interpretation of this statutory provision in a Warning Letter to Endotec Incorporated on March 15, 2002, as follows:

Among those requirements, a custom device must be intended for use by an individual patient named in a prescription and made in a special form for that patient or must be intended to meet the special needs of a particular health professional in the course of his professional practice. A special need is one that relates to unusual anatomical features of the individual physician for whom the device is produced, or to special needs of his or her practice that are not shared by other health professionals of the same specialty. A device that meets a need that is shared by others in the field is a device that can be tested through clinical investigations and can be subject to the PMA requirements in order to ensure that it is safe and effective. These requirements are to be narrowly construed and do not create an exemption from otherwise applicable statutory requirements.

PMA and Performance Standard Exemption

Custom devices are exempt from certain requirements of the FDCA. The Act extends a limited exemption to the mandatory performance standard requirements and the PMA requirements to devices that meet the definition of a custom device.

IDE and 510(k) Exemption

In addition to the statutory provision providing exemptions to a custom device, FDA, by regulation, also exempted a custom device from the requirements of the IDE and 510(k) regulations. Thus, it is not necessary to obtain an approved IDE or cleared 510(k) before shipment of the custom device in interstate commerce.

GMP Applicability

Custom devices, however, are not exempt from the GMP requirements. Current FDA policy, however, is to not inspect manufacturers of custom devices, but manufacturers of custom devices should comply with the GMP requirements.

Custom Device Litigation

A major difficulty arises, however, when a device is shipped in interstate commerce as a custom device and FDA takes the position that the device does not meet the definition of a custom device. It was this difference of opinion between Endotec, the company named in the Warning Letter above, and FDA that led to litigation.

PART 14. EXERCISES

1. What are the basic constitutional and statutory authorities for the regulation of medical devices in the United States?

2. Explain the differences between legal requirements and quasi-legal requirements, and name three types of each requirement that may be applicable to medical device design and development.

3. Search the FDA website and identify a level 1 guidance document and a level 2 guidance document. Briefly explain the essence of each one.

4. What are the three main steps in the promulgation of a regulation?

5. Identify the major bases for the overturn of an agency action by a court under judicial review.

6. Name the major types of information that industry and FDA consider to be confidential.

7. Name the three types of auditing that may be employed, when necessary, by a medical device manufacturer.

8. What are the three major classes of medical devices and the criteria for determining the class to which a device is assigned?

2
Medical Device Design

After conceptualization of a medical device, the next step in the development of the device is the design stage. Not only is it the next step, it may also be, in fact, the most important stage in device development; if the design is not correct, the device may be ineffective or unsafe, and it may not be approved for marketing by FDA.

A great deal of attention must be paid to device design, and there are multiple steps in the design stage that are critical to coming up with a well-designed device. These steps are so important that FDA has formalized the procedures that must be established and maintained to control all aspects of the design of the device in order to ensure that specified design requirements are met. Failure to meet the regulatory requirements during the design stage may result in a violative product subject to action by FDA. Even more importantly, the device may be a commercial flop due to its failure to perform properly or due to the harm it causes.

FDA's design control requirements are part of the Quality System Regulation (QSR). Design control requirements are extracted from the QSR for discussion here because device design represents the beginning of the device development process. The remainder of the QSR, dealing with good manufacturing practices, is discussed in Chapter 7, Quality Systems and GMPs.

FDA has provided guidance for industry and FDA staff on the design control requirements in the document *Design Control Guidance for Medical Device Manufacturers*, which can be found at:

http://www.fda.gov/MedicalDevices/DeviceRegulationand Guidance/GuidanceDocuments/ucm070627.htm

It is important to keep in mind that medical device design is not a new topic. Design control systems of varying sophistication have been in use for medical device development for many years. Not surprisingly, medical device design control has been the subject of voluntary standards developed by international organizations as an essential component of a quality assurance program for the development, production, installation, and servicing of medical devices. Two well-known international standards that are in widespread use are:

- *ISO 9001:2008 Quality management systems—Requirements*

- *ISO 13485:2003 Medical devices—Quality management systems—Requirements for regulatory purposes*

In addition, the Global Harmonization Task Force has been active since 1992 in trying to harmonize the various international regulatory requirements in place within different jurisdictions.

All of these influences were on the table when FDA developed its own Quality System Regulation, and the current QSR represents the best compromise in adopting a comprehensive approach to design control while at the same time minimizing conflicts with other standards and regulations.

For a comparison of the QSR with the previous versions of the foregoing standards, dated August 5, 2003, see:

http://elsmar.com/pdf_files/ISO-9001-2000-ISO-13485-2003-FDA-QSR-correspondence-matrix.pdf

PART 1. DESIGN CONTROL BACKGROUND

Section 1. Overview of Design Control

When Congress passed the Safe Medical Devices Act (SMDA) of 1990, it included, among its many provisions, the authority for FDA to add preproduction design controls to the Good Manufacturing Practice (GMP) regulation for medical devices. On June 1, 1997, the Quality System Regulation, including design controls, became effective.

Design Failures

Prior to the promulgation of the device design control regulations, it became apparent that many of the problems encountered in medical devices were due to failures during the design process. Some of the common deficiencies in the design of medical devices centered on insufficient characterization or description of the device and its operation due to inadequate or omitted control of:

- The design/engineering drawings of the device

- The rationale for the device's design

- The device and performance specifications

- The description of materials (including biocompatibility information)

- The description of the device's function—how the device, components, and subsystems work together to achieve the desired function

- The verification and validation testing for the subsystems and the main system

The extent of design failures was studied and documented by FDA and cited in the preamble to the Quality System Regulation in the *Federal Register* at 61 FR 52602 (October 7, 1996), where it states:

> ... in January 1990, FDA published the results of an evaluation of device recalls that occurred from October 1983 through September 1989, in a report entitled "Device Recalls: A Study of Quality Problems" ... (See 55 FR 21108, May 22, 1990, where FDA announced the availability of the report.) *FDA found that approximately 44 percent of the quality problems that led to voluntary recall actions during this 6-year period were attributed to errors or deficiencies that were designed into particular devices and may have been prevented by adequate design controls.* These design-related defects involved both noncritical devices (e.g., patient chair lifts, in vitro diagnostics, and administration sets) and critical devices (e.g., pacemakers and ventilators). Also in 1990, the Department of Health and Human Services' Inspector General conducted a study entitled "FDA Medical Device Regulation from Premarket Review to Recall" ... which reached similar conclusions. *With respect to software used to operate medical devices, the data were even more striking. A subsequent study of software-related recalls for the period of fiscal year (FY) 1983 through FY 1991 indicated that over 90 percent of all software-related device failures were due to design-related errors, generally, the failure to validate software prior to routine production ....* [Emphasis added.]

This information led Congress to authorize and the FDA to adopt design control requirements.

Purpose of the Design Control Regulation

Prior to the promulgation of the QSR, FDA had in place the 1978 GMPs, which did not include design control requirements. Pursuant to the authority granted by the SMDA, the 1997 QSR added design controls. The purposes of the design control requirements were to (1) establish and maintain procedures to control the design of the device, (2) establish the intrinsic quality of the device to assure that specified design requirements will meet user needs, the device's intended uses, and its specifications, (3) assure safety and effectiveness, and (4) reduce recalls.

Elements of FDA Design Control

The basic elements of a design control system include:

- Planning
- Design input
- Design output
- Design review
- Design verification
- Design validation
- Design transfer
- Design changes
- Design history file

In addition, risk analysis must be conducted for the majority of devices subject to design controls and is considered to be an essential requirement for medical devices under the regulation.

Management and Organizational Structure

The design control subsystem requires an appropriate management/organizational structure to assure that all design requirements have been met. FDA describes the need for this requirement in the QSR preamble at 61 FR 52613, where it states:

> . . . FDA has retained the requirement for establishing an "adequate organizational structure" to ensure compliance with the regulation, because such an organizational structure is fundamental to a manufacturer's ability to produce safe and effective devices. The organizational structure should ensure that the

technical, administrative, and human factors functions affecting the quality of the device will be controlled, whether these functions involve hardware, software, processed materials, or services. All such control should be oriented towards the reduction, elimination, or ideally, prevention of quality nonconformities. Further, the agency does not believe that the term is ambiguous. The organizational structure established will be determined in part by the type of device produced, the manufacturer's organizational goals, and the expectations and needs of customers. What may be an "adequate" organizational structure for manufacturing a relatively simple device may not be "adequate" for the production of a more complex device, such as a defibrillator.

Section 2. Applicability of FDA's Design Regulation

Device Classes Subject to Design Control Requirements

The design control requirements apply to all Class II and Class III devices, and to certain enumerated Class I devices. Device classification is discussed in Chapter 1, part 13, Medical Devices, Drugs, and Biologics.

Class I devices are not covered under the rationale stated by FDA in the QSR preamble, at 61 FR 52616, in the following way:

> FDA is not subjecting the majority of class I devices to design controls because FDA does not believe that such controls are necessary to ensure that such devices are safe and effective and otherwise in compliance with the act. However, all devices, including class I devices exempt from design controls, must be properly transferred to production in order to comply with Sec. 820.181, as well as other applicable requirements. For most class I devices, FDA believes that the production and other controls in the new quality system regulation and other general controls of the act will be sufficient, as they have been in the past, to ensure safety and effectiveness.

Based on this approach, the FDA regulations require design control for the following enumerated Class I devices.

- Devices automated with computer software

- Tracheobronchial suction catheters

- Surgeon's gloves

- Protective restraints

- Manual radionuclide applicator systems

- Radionuclide teletherapy sources

In addition to the foregoing, design controls also apply to preproduction stages and to the processing of "reuse" devices.

Design controls do not apply to concepts and feasibility studies. This raises the question of when to implement design controls. The regulation advises us that the requirements take effect when the development decision is made, which occurs when management decides that it is feasible to market the device and management decides to devote specific resources to design development.

FDA Inspection under Design Controls

It helps to know how FDA approaches the enforcement of design control requirements. FDA investigators will evaluate a manufacturer's processes, methods, and procedures to implement design controls, and they will report their findings to CDRH for review and action, if necessary. FDA investigators will not determine if the device is safe and effective based on the design control implementation. This can be a tricky decision point for management. It would not be a bad idea to have a memo in the design control records indicating the specific time when this decision was made and the basis for the decision. Such a memo could help avoid any dispute with FDA as to when the design control requirements became effective.

Section 3. International Design Control Standards

As stated in the introduction to this part, there are two major international standards dealing with device design as part of quality system requirements:

- *ISO 9001:2008 Quality management systems—Requirements*

- *ISO 13485:2003 Medical devices—Quality management systems—Requirements for regulatory purposes*

Device designers use these standards on a regular basis to assure that the design, in addition to the overall quality of the device, meets the generally recognized standards of the international community. These standards, like all standards, are subject to periodic revision, so it is important to be sure the latest versions are used.

PART 2. DESIGN PLANNING AND RECORD KEEPING

Section 1. Design Planning

Design planning has been described in *The FDA and Worldwide Quality System Requirements Guidebook for Medical Devices,* a book originally written by Kimberly Trautman, the GMP/quality systems expert at CDRH. It states, at page 55:

> The design plan typically includes the specific quality practices, assessment methodology, record keeping, documentation requirements, resources, etc., and sequence of activities relevant to a particular design or design category. The plan should reference applicable codes, standards, regulations, and specifications. However, the plan should only be as comprehensive as needed to meet the quality objectives.

Features of a Good Design Plan

Good design planning will establish and maintain design plans that describe the design and development activities. This road map will provide for, among other matters: sequential and parallel work schedules and timelines; design verification activities; evaluating safety, performance, and dependability; methods of measurement and testing; acceptance; and assignment of responsibilities. The plan should be reviewed, updated, and approved as design and development evolves. It will establish a *design history file* (DHF) or *device master record* (DMR) for design control documentation. In addition, the plan should establish and maintain plans that describe or reference design and development activities, define responsibility for implementation, and identify or describe interfaces with different groups or activities. Lastly, the plan should provide for the review, updating, and approval as design and development evolves.

Contents of the Plan

The design plan should contain the goals, objectives, and scope of the design stage. In doing so it would identify and describe the major tasks and deliverables, all schedules, available resources and assignment of responsibilities, the details of who will review the design activities, when the reviews will take place, and how design issues will be tracked. It must also identify the individuals who are authorized to approve the various stages of device design.

The Life Span of the Design Plan

A design plan is a living document. After the design is adopted and the device moves on to the subsequent development, manufacturing, and marketing phases, the design plan may still come into play. During the non-clinical and clinical testing of the device, the verification and validation of the device may necessitate a change in the design of the device. During the transfer of the design to the manufacturing process, it may become evident that the design is in need of a change. When a post-approval study is required, long-term data may reveal yet another change that must be undertaken in the device design. Based on post-market complaints from users, a subsequent recall and corrective and preventive action plan may uncover additional device modifications that are necessary. Under any of these circumstances that occur after the initial design is adopted, the need to make changes to the original design plan may arise. In this manner, the design plan may come alive at any time.

Each of the conditions identified above are discussed in later chapters, and it will become evident that the design effort does not necessarily end after the final device design is adopted, and will potentially be "in play" for the useful life of the device.

Section 2. Design History File

A major component of design planning and management is the *design history file* (DHF). This file should contain the complete design history of a finished device. QSR requires that the device designer establish and maintain a DHF for each type of device. The DHF should contain, for example, the design and development plan, design review results, design verification results, and design validation results, as well as any other data necessary to establish compliance with the design requirements. The DHF also may contain references to these records.

The designer must also establish standard operating procedures for the control of all documents required by the regulation dealing with document approval and distribution and document changes.

The DHF should also contain all of the design records, or references to the records, as required under each of the design control functions discussed elsewhere in this chapter. This requirement is explained in the QSR preamble, at 61 FR 52622:

> The DHF . . . contains or references all the records necessary to establish compliance with the design plan and the regulation, including the design control procedures. The DHF illustrates the history of the design, and is necessary so that manufacturers can

exercise control over and be accountable for the design process, thereby maximizing the probability that the finished design conforms to the design specifications.

These requirements are applicable to all phases of design control, and should be implemented. In addition to design control documentation, following chapters discuss information about additional documentation and record keeping that is particularly related to the function under discussion in those chapters.

PART 3. DESIGN INPUTS AND OUTPUTS

Section 1. Design Inputs

Basic Requirements for Design Inputs

In promulgating the design input requirements, FDA made clear that it intended the design inputs to be consistent with previously established standards and with the needs of the human interfacing that will occur. It went on to describe in the QSR preamble, at 61 FR 52618, what the regulation required:

> . . . FDA emphasizes, however, that the section requires the manufacturer to ensure that the design input requirements are appropriate so the device will perform to meet its intended use and the needs of the user. In doing this, the manufacturer must define the performance characteristics, safety and reliability requirements, environmental requirements and limitations, physical characteristics, applicable standards and regulatory requirements, and labeling and packaging requirements, among other things, and refine the design requirements as verification and validation results are established. For example, when designing a device, the manufacturer should conduct appropriate human factors studies, analyses, and tests from the early stages of the design process until that point in development at which the interfaces with the medical professional and the patient are fixed. The human interface includes both the hardware and software characteristics that affect device use, and good design is crucial to logical, straightforward, and safe device operation. The human factors methods used (for instance, task/function analyses, user studies, prototype tests, mock-up reviews, etc.) should ensure that the characteristics of the user

population and operating environment are considered. In addition, the compatibility of system components should be assessed. Finally, labeling (e.g., instructions for use) should be tested for usability. FDA emphasizes, however, that the section requires the manufacturer to ensure that the design input requirements are appropriate so the device will perform to meet its intended use and the needs of the user. In doing this, the manufacturer must define the performance characteristics, safety and reliability requirements, environmental requirements and limitations, physical characteristics, applicable standards and regulatory requirements, and labeling and packaging requirements, among other things, and refine the design requirements as verification and validation results are established.

The preparation of design inputs generally requires consideration and definition of relevant characteristics and design requirements related to the intended use of the device, the needs of the user, the needs of the patient, and the methods for resolving incomplete, ambiguous, or conflicting requirements.

Inputs should be expressed in terms that are measurable. For example, if the device should be portable, what does "portable" mean? How is it defined and measured?

Also, design inputs require documentation that is signed and dated by an approving individual.

Examples of Design Inputs

The following items are examples of what should be considered when identifying design inputs.

- Applicable standards
- Regulatory requirements
- Labeling requirements
- Packaging requirements
- Human factors
- MDRs and complaints
- Customers
- Competitors' products
- Performance characteristics

- Safety and reliability requirements

- Environmental requirements and limitations

- Physical characteristics

- Service reports

- Marketing surveys

Examples of basic, yet essential, sources of design inputs and the information each would supply for a 510(k) device include:

- Classification regulations

  - Official name

  - Class I, II, or III

  - Classification code

  - The classification regulations can be searched at: http://www.accessdata.fda.gov/scripts/cdrh/cfdocs/cfPCD/classification.cfm

- Clearance documents for similar 510(k) devices

  - Description of the device

  - Device specifications

  - Form factor

  - Materials

  - Cleared 510(k)s can be searched at: http://www.accessdata.fda.gov/scripts/cdrh/cfdocs/cfpmn/pmn.cfm

- Recalls/Warning Letters

  - Identification of problems encountered in similar devices

  - Identification of and solutions for problems to factor into the design

  - Recalls are found at: http://www.fda.gov/MedicalDevices/Safety/RecallsCorrectionsRemovals/ListofRecalls/default.htm

  - Warning Letters are published at: http://www.fda.gov/ICECI/EnforcementActions/WarningLetters/default.htm

- FDA's *Patient Safety News.* The PSN website is: http://www.accessdata.fda.gov/scripts/cdrh/cfdocs/psn/index.cfm

Patient Safety News is discussed below in part 7, Design Failures. The classification regulations were discussed in Chapter 1, part 13, Medical Devices, Drugs, and Biologics; 510(k)s are discussed in Chapter 5, part 2, Premarket Notification (510[k]); recalls are included in Chapter 6, part 4, Medical Device Recalls; and Warning Letters are covered in Chapter 8, part 2, Compliance Actions and Penalties.

Types of Design Inputs

The specific inputs, in measurable terms, that should appear in the design plan would include the following items:

- Device functions

- Physical characteristics

- Performance

- Safety

- Reliability

- Environmental limits

- Labeling

- Human factors

- Maintenance

- Compatibility with other devices

- Sterility

Section 2. Human Factors Engineering

Medical devices are designed and intended for use in the treatment of human beings. It is not surprising, therefore, that human factors engineering (HFE) is critical and a major component in designing a medical device. HFE involves hardware and software studies, analyses, and tests to assure proper interfaces with the healthcare professional and the patient. The goal is logical, straightforward, and safe device operation in the user population and operating environment.

Factors that must be considered relate to user population characteristics, energy sources (electrical, heat, electromagnetic fields), biological effects (toxicity and biocompatibility), and environmental effects (electromagnetic interference, electrostatic discharge). Also, labeling should be tested for usability. FDA identified many elements and methods used in HFE. See the comprehensive discussion by FDA as quoted in section 1 above.

Section 3. Design Outputs

The design outputs stage establishes the measurements that will determine whether the design inputs have been met. FDA describes design outputs in the following manner in the QSR preamble at 61 FR 52619:

> Design outputs are the design specifications which should meet design input requirements, as confirmed during design verification and validation and ensured during design review. The output includes the device, its labeling and packaging, associated specifications and drawings, and production and quality assurance specifications and procedures.

Meeting the design outputs means that the results of a design effort, at each design phase and at the end of the total design effort, are successful. The total finished design outputs consist of the device, its packaging and labeling, and the device master record.

The design outputs plan should identify acceptable criteria to ensure that the device will function properly, and document the procedures that will allow adequate evaluation of conformance to design input requirements.

There should be standard operating procedures (SOPs) for defining and documenting design outputs in terms that allow an adequate evaluation of conformance to design inputs requirements, containing or referencing acceptance criteria, and ensuring design outputs essential for the proper functioning of the device.

Documenting Design Outputs

The finished design outputs are the basis for the device master record. The designated individual(s) must document, review, and approve design outputs before release. The approving individual(s) must date and sign the outputs.

PART 4. DESIGN VERIFICATION AND DESIGN VALIDATION

For those medical devices to which design controls apply, the design of the device must be verified and validated. It is important to distinguish between design verification and validation:

- *Design verification* means confirmation by examination and provision of objective evidence that specified requirements have been fulfilled. In other words, did I make the product right?
- *Design validation* means establishing by objective evidence that device specifications conform to user needs and intended uses. In this case, the question to be answered is, did I make the right product?

Each of these is discussed separately below. Although there are similarities in the approach and implementation of each of these processes, it is important to know how they differ and when each may be permissible or required. To paraphrase FDA's statement in the QSR preamble at 61 FR 52620:

> It is important to note that although design validation follows successful design verification, certain aspects of design validation can be accomplished during the design verification. Nevertheless, design verification is not a substitute for design validation.

Section 1. Verification

The ISO international standard ISO 8402:1994 states that verification consists of:

> . . . information which can be proved true, based on facts obtained through observation, measurement, test, or other means.

Design verification is intended to ensure that you built the device you designed in accordance with its specifications, that is, did you build it right? It involves procedures to verify that the design outputs meet the design inputs requirements. To know when verification, as opposed to validation, is adequate for the design feature, the FDA QSR preamble advises, at 61 FR 52622:

> FDA . . . permit(s) verification where appropriate. For example, a change in the sterilization process of a catheter will require validation of the new process, but the addition of more chromium to a stainless steel surgical instrument may only require verification through chemical analysis. Where a design change cannot be verified by subsequent inspection and test, it must be validated.

Verification Records

The results of the design verification must be documented in the DHF, including the identification of the design, a description of the methods of design verification, and the date and name of the individual(s) performing verification. Verification requires documentation that is signed and dated by an approving individual.

Section 2. Validation

Definition of Design Validation

There are two major types of validation that come into play with medical devices—design validation and process validation:

- *Design validation* means establishing, by objective evidence, that device specifications conform to the user's needs and the device's intended uses.

- *Process validation* means establishing, by objective evidence, that a process consistently produces the desired result or a product meeting the predetermined specifications.

General Design Validation

In order to conduct proper design validation, it is important to establish and maintain written procedures for this purpose. The design validation should be performed under defined operating conditions under actual or simulated use conditions. The procedures should include software validation and risk analysis, where appropriate, and be conducted on the initial production units, lots, or batches, or their equivalents, to ensure proper overall design control and proper design transfer. As with all other aspects of a design control system, there must be documentation that is signed and dated by an approving individual.

Risk Analysis

When conducting a risk analysis, manufacturers are expected to identify possible hazards associated with the design in both normal and fault conditions, including those resulting from user error. Unacceptable risks should be reduced to acceptable levels. This may require redesigning the device or changing the manufacturing process. Some risks may be reduced through appropriate warnings. An important part of risk analysis is ensuring that changes made to eliminate or minimize hazards do not introduce new hazards. Two tools suggested by FDA for this purpose are *failure mode and effects analysis* and *fault tree analysis,* but there are others as well.

Software Validation

Software validation is a very specialized area. FDA has specialists who deal with software validation. FDA guidance for industry and staff on software validation can be found at:

http://www.fda.gov/downloads/MedicalDevices/Device
RegulationandGuidance/GuidanceDocuments/UCM085371.pdf

Prototypes, Finished Devices, and Equivalent Devices

Validation may occur during any stage of development from concept to
finished product. The FDA distinguishes between conducting validation
testing on prototypes, finished devices, and equivalent devices in the manner stated in the QSR preamble at 61 FR 52620.

Prototypes

Manufacturers should not use prototypes developed in the laboratory or machine shop as test units to meet these requirements. Prototypes may differ from the finished production devices. During
research and development, conditions for building prototypes are
typically better controlled and personnel more knowledgeable
about what needs to be done and how to do it than are regular production personnel. When going from laboratory to scale-up
production, standards, methods, and procedures may not be
properly transferred, or additional manufacturing processes may
be added. Often, changes not reflected in the prototype are made
in the device to facilitate the manufacturing process, and these
may adversely affect device functioning and user interface characteristics. Proper testing of devices that are produced using the
same methods and procedures as those to be used in routine production will prevent the distribution and subsequent recall of many
unacceptable medical devices.

Finished Devices

In addition, finished devices must be tested for performance under
actual conditions of use or simulated use conditions in the actual
or simulated environment in which the device is expected to be
used. The simulated use testing provision no longer requires that
the testing be performed on the *first three* production runs. However, samples must be taken from units, lots, or batches that were
produced using the same specifications, production and quality
system methods, procedures, and equipment that will be used
for routine production. FDA considers this a critical element of
the design validation. The requirement to conduct simulated use
testing of finished devices is found in the original CGMP in Sec.
820.160, as part of finished device inspection. This requirement
has been moved to Sec. 820.30(g) because FDA believes that

simulated use testing at this point is more effective in ensuring that only safe and effective devices are produced.

Equivalent Devices

When equivalent devices are used in the final design validation, the manufacturer must document in detail how the device was manufactured and how the manufacturing is similar to and possibly different from initial production. Where there are differences, the manufacturer must justify why design validation results are valid for the production units, lots, or batches.

PART 5. DESIGN REVIEW AND DOCUMENTATION

The purpose of conducting a design review is to ensure that the design satisfies the design inputs requirements for the intended use of the device and the needs of the user. *Design review* means a documented, comprehensive, systematic examination of a design to evaluate the adequacy of the design requirements, to evaluate the capability of the design to meet these requirements, and to identify problems.

This review can take place at various times during the development process. The review provides information that may be used to loop back to an earlier design stage and make necessary changes to the design. The FDA provides a schematic to illustrate the feedback process of design review, which is presented in Figure 2.1.

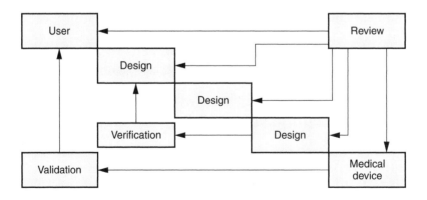

Figure 2.1 Design and review process.

The number of design reviews will depend on the plan and the complexity of the device. Multiple reviews can occur, and the manufacturer must document what is being reviewed, when, and by whom.

Design Review Plan

The design review plan should provide for formal documented reviews, identify the timing of reviews, and describe what procedures will be used and which specialists will conduct the review of specific functions of the design.

The plan must have at least one independent reviewer not responsible for the design function being reviewed, and any specialists that may be needed. It requires documentation that is signed and dated by an approving individual, and the results of design review must be documented in the design history file.

Design Verification Review

Design review includes the review of design verification data to determine whether:

- The design outputs meet functional and operational requirements

- The design is compatible with components and other accessories

- The safety requirements are achieved

- The reliability and maintenance requirements are met

- The labeling and other regulatory requirements are met

- The manufacturing, installation, and servicing requirements are compatible with the design specifications

Design Control Relationships

Designers use many different techniques and instruments for managing and reviewing the design control process such as program evaluation and review technique (PERT) charts, flowcharts, and other project management tools. Taking all of the elements of design control into account, it is possible to construct a relational table that ties these principles together. Figure 2.2 is a representation of how the inputs, outputs, verification, validation, and design review relate to each other. It should be possible to track each characteristic or value of a device from the input all the way through to the final review and acceptance. This enables managers to assure that all of the required steps for the control of a design are logical and have been completed satisfactorily.

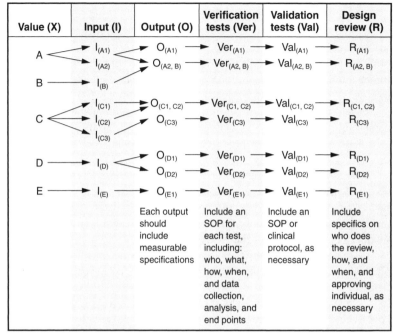

Value (X)	Input (I)	Output (O)	Verification tests (Ver)	Validation tests (Val)	Design review (R)
A	$I_{(A1)}$ $I_{(A2)}$	$O_{(A1)}$ $O_{(A2, B)}$	$Ver_{(A1)}$ $Ver_{(A2, B)}$	$Val_{(A1)}$ $Val_{(A2, B)}$	$R_{(A1)}$ $R_{(A2, B)}$
B	$I_{(B)}$				
C	$I_{(C1)}$ $I_{(C2)}$ $I_{(C3)}$	$O_{(C1, C2)}$ $O_{(C3)}$	$Ver_{(C1, C2)}$ $Ver_{(C3)}$	$Val_{(C1, C2)}$ $Val_{(C3)}$	$R_{(C1, C2)}$ $R_{(C3)}$
D	$I_{(D)}$	$O_{(D1)}$ $O_{(D2)}$	$Ver_{(D1)}$ $Ver_{(D2)}$	$Val_{(D1)}$ $Val_{(D2)}$	$R_{(D1)}$ $R_{(D2)}$
E	$I_{(E)}$	$O_{(E1)}$	$Ver_{(E1)}$	$Val_{(E1)}$	$R_{(E1)}$
		Each output should include measurable specifications	Include an SOP for each test, including: who, what, how, when, and data collection, analysis, and end points	Include an SOP or clinical protocol, as necessary	Include specifics on who does the review, how, when, and approving individual, as necessary

Figure 2.2   Design control relationships.

PART 6. DESIGN TRANSFER AND DESIGN CHANGES

Section 1. Design Transfer

Design transfer requires the establishment and maintenance of SOPs to ensure that the device design is correctly translated into production specifications. Manufacturers have an interest in beginning the production process as soon as possible so the process transfer moves along as efficiently as possible. However, FDA requires that all design specifications released to production have been approved, verified, and validated before they are implemented as part of the production process.

Section 2. Design Changes

Design change is a healthy and necessary part of product development. However, quality can be ensured only if change is controlled and documented in the development process, as well as the production process.

To accomplish this goal, SOPs for dealing with design changes must be adopted to ensure that changes to the design, both preproduction and post-production, are also reviewed, validated (or verified where appropriate), and approved. These procedures must provide for the identification, documentation, validation, or, where appropriate, verification, review, and approval of design changes before their implementation.

In addition to the SOPs, the manufacturer must establish criteria for evaluating changes to ensure that the changes are appropriate for its designs. Otherwise, a device may be rendered unable to properly perform, and this failure may render the device unsafe or ineffective.

Design change requirements apply to any preproduction changes to the device design or changes made in the manufacturing process, including packaging and labeling. They also apply to changes made after the device has been marketed. Changes must be controlled whether they occur during the development process or the production process.

Change control requirements apply, and testing must be conducted when the manufacturer makes changes in the device design or the manufacturing process that could affect safety or effectiveness. The extent of testing conducted should be governed by the risks the device will present if it fails. This assures that the manufacturing process does not adversely affect the device. See the discussion of risk analysis above in part 4, Design Verification and Design Validation.

Lastly, it should be noted that where a design change can not be verified by subsequent inspection and testing, it must be validated.

Section 3. Documentation of Design Change

A device may undergo many changes during the developmental stage of device design. Manufacturers are not expected to maintain records of all changes proposed during the very early stages of the design process. The change control requirements and the need for documentation become effective with respect to all design changes made after the design review that approves the initial design inputs, and those changes made to correct design deficiencies once the design has been released to production.

The amount of documentation may vary from change to change. The agency advises that the evaluation and documentation should be in direct proportion to the significance of the change. The intent and purpose of these change records is to create a history of the evolution of the design, which can be invaluable for failure investigation and for facilitating the design of future similar products. Such records can prevent the repetition of errors and the development of unsafe or ineffective designs.

PART 7. DESIGN FAILURES

Now that each of the aspects of a good design control system has been discussed in the previous parts of this chapter, it is instructional to take a look at examples of design failures. In designing a new medical device or changes to an existing device, it can be helpful, some would say essential, to monitor known failures in marketed devices. The identification of design inputs listed above in part 3 includes many excellent sources of information about device failures. Take, for example, the last item in the list above. The FDA *Patient Safety News (PSN)* is a video news show for professionals and is available on the agency website at:

http://www.accessdata.fda.gov/scripts/cdrh/cfdocs/psn/index.cfm

The show can be watched, or the transcripts of each show can be read. The *PSN* covers many diverse topics related to the safe use of medical devices. Identification of these problems can be important as a source of inputs for device design actions. The multiple problems that have been found in medical device use may relate, for example, to materials, durability, method of use, and human factors engineering considerations, including adequate instructions for use. The following examples of design failures come from different sources, as indicated.

Design Failure—Example 1

The *PSN* program for June 2010 includes a news item based on an article in the journal *Nursing 2010*. That article describes adverse events that have occurred during use of temporary pacing leads. The following three examples from that article on pacing leads are instructional:

- *Inadvertent disconnections.* A new reusable extension cable was provided that was supposed to connect the lead to the pacemaker. In many cases the new cable would inadvertently disconnect. This did not happen with the original cable.

- *Lead fractures.* The distal tip of a temporary epicardial lead broke off and remained in the patient when the lead was removed 13 days after surgery. The lead manufacturer had recommended only a seven-day implant duration.

- *Misconnections.* In another case, IV tubing was accidentally connected to the pacing catheter's balloon inflation port, causing the balloon to burst inside the patient.

Each of these problems has to be looked upon as a potential design failure. These adverse events raise the following, as well as other, design issues:

- Could not better verification and validation testing have uncovered the defects encountered and prevented injury to these patients?

- Could better user testing of the labeling identify the need to include an enhanced warning about not implanting the lead for more than seven days?

- Would better nonclinical testing of the distal tip have prevented its breaking?

Answering these types of questions could result in better design control outcomes in the device development process.

Design Failure—Example 2

On July 9, 2010, FDA issued an open letter to manufacturers of enteral feeding tubes, healthcare professionals, and hospital purchasing departments concerning problems with standard Luer lock connectors. Luer locks are used primarily in institutions along with, and as part of, other complex devices. Thus, the letter covers many aspects of design issues, user methods, and post-market modifications and is worthy of consideration when discussing device design. Set forth below are extracts from that letter:

> FDA is aware that standard Luer lock connectors are found on a variety of tubing sets, solution bags, and other medical products. The ease of connection between these Luer lock connectors have *[sic]* led to misconnections that have inadvertently linked unrelated systems, and at times, have resulted in serious adverse events. Luer lock misconnections are often under-recognized; therefore, adverse events resulting from such misconnections are likely to be under-reported.
>
> . . .
>
> Luer connectors easily interconnect many medical components, accessories, and delivery systems across multiple medical applications. Because of the nature of the connector design, human factors, and the clinical environment, healthcare professionals may mistakenly connect the wrong devices and deliver substances through the wrong route.
>
> Examples of misconnections include:
>
> - Intravenous infusions connected to epidural lines, and epidural solutions (intended for epidural administration) connected to peripheral or central IV catheters.

- Bladder irrigation solutions using primary intravenous tubing connected as secondary infusions to peripheral or central IV catheters.

- Infusions intended for IV administration connected to an indwelling bladder (foley) catheter.

- Infusions intended for IV administration connected to nasogastric (NG) tubes.

- Intravenous solutions administered with blood administration sets, and blood products transfused with primary intravenous tubing.

- Primary intravenous solutions administered through various other functionally dissimilar catheters, such as external dialysis catheters, a ventriculostomy drain, an amnio-infusion catheter, and the distal port of a pulmonary artery catheter.

In particular, misconnections with enteral feeding tubes and solutions have been associated with death and serious injury. Although these adverse events appear to occur at a low frequency, it is suspected that many misconnections are recorded as medication errors.

To address this problem, the letter has the following design recommendations for manufacturers:

To reduce the likelihood of errors, some manufacturers have implemented design changes. For example, some have chosen to color-code and label their enteral feeding tubes to flag which tubes must be connected with one another. Others have opted to create proprietary connections, following the principle of designed incompatibility, to ensure that devices that should not be connected cannot, in fact, be connected.

FDA believes manufacturers should provide the necessary safeguards to ensure safe use of these devices and products. We encourage all manufacturers to assess the risks of misconnections for these devices, carefully consider both temporary and long-term options to mitigate the risk, and validate the solution(s) they deem most appropriate. FDA will assess the validation of the proposed solution during the course of the premarket review, as appropriate.

The letter also has suggestions for healthcare professionals using these devices in the institutional setting:

Healthcare professionals can institute practices such as, but not limited to:

- Not modifying or adapting devices since that may defeat the safety system;

- Tracing lines back to its *[sic]* origins when reconnecting devices;

- Routing tubes and catheters that have different purposes in unique and standardized directions.

Lastly, the letter provides information about the use of standards to address the Luer lock design issues:

The current Association for the Advancement of Medical Instrumentation/American National Standards Institute, Inc. (AAMI/ANSI) standard, ID54:1996/(R)2005 entitled "Enteral feeding set adapters and connectors" recommends that adapters provided with, or are for use with, enteral feeding sets be designed so that they are incompatible with rigid Luer connectors. However, this standard does not set out any specifications for these adapters.

FDA wants to inform you that a new broad-ranging standard is currently under development: ISO/IEC/FDIS 80369-1, "Small-bore connectors for liquids and gases in healthcare applications." This standard, and the series of standards that will accompany it, are intended to address connector cross-compatibility issues between products used for a variety of medical applications (e.g., enteral, parenteral, IV, epidural, etc.), and will likely identify specific designs for each application to eliminate the possibility of misconnections. FDA is actively participating in the development of the standard and believes this standard will help prevent device misconnections through, for example, the use of force function design and usability testing. FDA is considering recognizing this standard when it is published. If FDA recognizes the standard, due to the significant impact this standard may likely have on the safety of these devices, FDA will provide guidance to manufacturers regarding issues such as whether there will be a set period of time for currently marketed devices to come into compliance and the effect of the standard on new devices.

This letter may be read in its entirety at:

http://www.fda.gov/downloads/MedicalDevices/Resourcesfor
You/Industry/UCM218631.pdf

PART 8. EXERCISES

1. Identify the major elements of a medical device design control
   plan that is in compliance with FDA regulatory requirements.

2. At what point in the development of a medical device do the FDA
   design regulations become applicable?

3. To what classes of devices do the design control requirements
   apply?

4. Prepare a list of the types of deficiencies in the design stage of a
   medical device that can lead to device failures.

5. In your opinion, what is the most important element of a good
   device design plan? Please explain why.

6. You are the director of research and development for the Perfect
   Vision Innovations Corporation. The president tells you that the
   board of directors loves your idea for a new daily wear soft contact
   lens. She asks you to prepare, for presentation to the board, a
   proposed design control and development plan for the new contact
   lens. Please prepare this plan and accompanying slides for the
   presentation.

7. You are a biomedical engineer for a firm that is designing medical
   devices for use by astronauts on their upcoming voyage to Mars.
   Due to weight and size restrictions of the voyager, the crew will
   not include a physician or nurse, so the astronauts will have to
   provide healthcare to each other during the mission. You have
   been assigned to work on the development of an automated
   external defibrillator (AED) for use by the astronauts if the need
   arises. Explain how you will use the principles of human factors
   engineering to assure that the astronauts will be able to properly
   use it in outer space for its intended uses.

8. List five examples of sources of design inputs.

9. List five examples of types of design inputs.

10. Explain the differences between design verification and design validation.

11. What is the purpose of design verification review?

12. Search the FDA Warning Letters database and identify three Warning Letters that contain deficiencies arising out of inadequate design controls. In a report identify, for each letter, the company name and date and quote the deficiency. Explain what you would do to correct the deficiency and prevent it from happening again.

3

Nonclinical Testing and GLPs

Nonclinical testing encompasses any type of testing other than clinical trials involving human subjects. Such testing may take place in a laboratory within a device manufacturer's facility, in an off-site contract testing laboratory, or in an animal test facility.

Examples of the types of testing that may be conducted during the nonclinical testing phase include mechanical, sterility, biocompatibility, stability, and animal testing. It could also include electrical safety testing, software validation testing, and chemical testing. The exact tests that will be required depend on the structure, materials, functions, and intended uses of the device.

Data collected during this testing may be necessary to establish the substantial equivalency of the test device to a predicate device or to establish the suitability of the device for clinical trials. Thus, the test data may be necessary in a 510(k) submission, a PMA application, or an IDE application. The data would be submitted to FDA in the appropriate premarket submission for review and evaluation. IDE requirements are discussed in Chapter 4, part 5, Investigational Device Exemptions, and 510(k)s and PMAs are discussed in detail in Chapter 5, Marketing Applications.

PART 1. NONCLINICAL TESTING

Nonclinical testing consists of all tests conducted except for clinical trials using human subjects. Clinical trials and clinical protocols are discussed in Chapter 4, Clinical Trials. Some of the major purposes for conducting nonclinical tests are: to obtain an adequate description of a device, to gather comparative data on which the FDA can make a determination of substantial equivalency, or to gather sufficient test data to support an IDE approval to move on to clinical trials.

Section 1. General Principles

Medical device nonclinical testing is subject to the same general principles of good scientific practice as any other scientific testing. The following principles would be applicable to nonclinical testing, both laboratory and animal testing, of a medical device. They would also be applicable to clinical testing as well. These principles are identified in Table 3.1.

Those Who Need Standard Operating Procedures

Anyone who conducts nonclinical testing of a medical device to gather data that will be submitted to FDA, whether it is for laboratory testing or animal testing, will need standard operating procedures (SOPs) or protocols governing the testing.

It may be noted at this point that FDA requires these instruments for virtually all of the activities carried out in the design, development, testing, production, and post-market follow-up of a medical device. SOPs are used to control the systems and activities at all levels of the medical device development, manufacture, and distribution system, which includes device manufacturers, distributors, testing laboratories, clinical test sites, and user facilities. In other words, any regulated party should develop the necessary SOPs depending on and related to the functions they perform. Accordingly, SOPs are discussed in many other chapters of the book.

Section 2. SOPs and Protocols

FDA may inspect, review, evaluate, request changes to, and inspect any SOP or protocol as it deems necessary.

Form and Content of a Standard Operating Procedure

SOPs for nonclinical testing may take on different forms and contain different information depending on the company or testing facility and the purpose and use of the SOP. See sample SOP in Figure 3.1. SOPs usually contain some or all of the following elements, as well as others as may be needed for the particular testing being conducted:

- Title

- Control and version numbers

- Who prepared and who approved the SOP

- Where the SOP is to be located

- Where the SOP is contained in records

- The purpose of the SOP and rationale of why the test is appropriate

Table 3.1 Principles applicable to nonclinical and clinical medical device testing.

Establish the hypothesis	Clearly identify the purpose of the testing. Is the testing being conducted simply to establish the identity of the device, to show feasibility to proceed to clinical testing, to gather data to establish substantial equivalence, or to provide reasonable evidence of safety and effectiveness?
Establish appropriate acceptance criteria	The expected laboratory outputs, animal outcomes, or clinical results must be established, against which to measure the success of the testing. If the device is to be tested for substantial equivalence, identify the specifications and definition of the predicate device. If the device is to be tested in a subsequent clinical trial for safety and effectiveness, it may be necessary to develop a protocol for animal testing that will establish whether the device is appropriate for human testing. For a clinical trial, it is necessary to establish the primary and secondary end points.
Prepare appropriate SOPs for laboratory testing, and protocols for animal and clinical testing	All nonclinical testing should be conducted in accordance with an established operating procedure. Animal testing should be conducted per an acceptable testing protocol. The clinical testing also will require a clinical protocol.
Test the final device	It is preferable, and sometimes absolutely necessary, to use the final or production model of the device for testing. A preproduction model or components of the device may be used if they are the same in all critical aspects as the finished product. This similarity is required if conclusions are to be drawn about the final device from the testing of the preproduction model. Otherwise, the final production device must be used.
Gather and document test results	The test results should be well documented in lab notebooks or computer feeds for nonclinical testing. Clinical data should be recorded in each subject's medical record and on case report forms. The records should be dated and signed by the tester, and reviewed and accepted by an authorized individual.
Conduct an analysis	The data should be analyzed using an appropriate statistical technique.
Draw reasonable conclusions	Based on the statistical analysis, appropriate conclusions may be drawn from the test results.

New Medical Device Company
[Name of Nonclinical Test Procedure]

Control Information

Control number: Version number:

Prepared by: Date of SOP:

Department:

Location of SOP:

Date of testing:

SOP Test Requirements

Purpose/objective of the testing (rationale of test and relationship to the device use):

Equipment/instrumentation (diagrams of test setup):

Supplies/material/reagents:

Skill level of personnel performing tests:

Steps in the procedure/process (test conditions/sample size/duration):

Expected outcomes/pass/fail criteria with justifications:

Data Gathering, including deviations or failures:

Analysis/statistics to be used (relationship to expected clinical use):

Signature of person performing test and date of testing:

Signature of approving individual, title, and date:

Figure 3.1   Sample operating procedure for nonclinical testing.

- An identification of the equipment or instrumentation required for a test procedure, including diagrams of test setup, as necessary, and hardware and software versions

- A listing of the supplies, materials, and reagents needed

- The type of personnel that will perform the function

- The steps in the procedure or process, test conditions, duration of test, and so on

- Outcomes, if necessary, including pass/fail criteria, analysis/ statistics to be used, and the relationship to expected clinical use

- Signature of preparer and date of preparation

- Signature of approving individual and date of approval

Types of Protocols

There are two primary types of protocols that are used in the testing of a medical device: an animal testing protocol and a clinical trial protocol. Animal testing protocols are discussed below under part 2, Good Laboratory Practices. Clinical protocols are discussed in detail in Chapter 4, Clinical Trials.

Section 3. Device Description

General Considerations

A complete and accurate description of the device is essential to the proper evaluation of a device. The device description will consist of gathering enough data to demonstrate the various properties unique to the specific device design. FDA clears or approves devices based on their intended use, so the technological characteristics of the device should be consistent with the indications for use.

Furthermore, FDA clears or approves *devices,* not the materials used to make the device. While the materials and composition of the device will be important, the qualifications of the finished device will be the main determining factor in FDA's decision making.

One of the most basic elements in characterizing a device is the engineering drawings. These will be important to establish the physical structure and form factor of the device.

It is necessary to clearly establish the composition of the device and its components. A device may be composed of various metallic alloys, plastics, natural or synthetic biomaterials, or a composite material. Laboratory testing may be used to identify any incompatibilities between and among the different components of the device.

Depending on the composition, the materials may be degradable or nondegradable. If the former is true, a degradation profile and the degradation mechanism will influence the test requirements and the test setup. Where systems of devices are used, such as those in the orthopedic device area, it would be necessary to provide a clear identification of each existing component with which the new component (for example, a hip stem) may be mated (for example, femoral head and acetabular component).

Combination Products

For combination products, additional concerns arise that may require other specialized testing. Many combination products consist of a device and a drug or a biological product. The purpose of the device component in such a combination may provide the primary use, with the other product serving an adjunctive use. In other cases, the device may serve the secondary role as a vehicle for delivery of the drug or biologic. In either case, compatibility between the various products must be tested. For timed-release usage, elution testing will be called for. Combination products and examples are also discussed in Chapter 1, part 13, section 8, Combination Products.

Data Requirements

The kind and quantity of test data required will depend on the device, its intended use, and the type of premarket submission required. The testing would ordinarily be done in a step-by-step fashion. If the engineering test data are insufficient to support the necessary submission to FDA, then animal data may be necessary. If that is not sufficient to appropriately address agency concerns, then clinical testing may have to be undertaken.

Complete reports of the testing should be prepared, including detailed descriptions of the test setups, such as the apparatus used, the materials, devices tested, and the test conditions. The report should include, in addition to the results and conclusions, any deviations or failures, along with the rationale as to why such deviations or failures were not an issue. This should include worst-case justifications or rationales for the samples tested.

Finite element analysis (FEA), when it is appropriate to use in lieu of mechanical testing, would need to be justified and validated. As an example, see the discussion of this in the FDA guidance "Non-Clinical Information for Femoral Stem Prostheses," which can be found at:

http://www.fda.gov/MedicalDevices/DeviceRegulationand
Guidance/GuidanceDocuments/ucm071275.htm

Section 4. Performance Testing

Performance testing may include electromagnetic compatibility, electrical safety, reliability, and software functionality. In performance testing, the comparison of properties to an appropriate control can be important and sometimes necessary. When including these types of tests in a submission to FDA, it is important to include complete test reports.

Mechanical integrity testing may be required depending on the type of device involved, especially for a device that will experience stresses during use. FDA is particularly concerned about the durability of an implant to withstand expected *in vivo* static and dynamic loads. It is often challenging to justify loading and to characterize mechanical parameters with *in vitro* testing because the results are so dependent on the environment in which the device is used. It is also challenging to characterize use and reliability phenomena over time, especially for degradables. In such testing it may be necessary to increase the number of animals used in these studies in order to obtain a sufficient sample size to produce statistical significance.

Special Cases of Nonclinical Testing

Some devices are of particular concern to FDA. Generally, these are devices that can play a critical role in the health and well-being of the patient, or those that present a potentially serious risk to the patient. This may also include devices that present difficult or unique issues that require special testing before FDA can adequately review the submission. In many such cases, FDA has issued a guidance document for the information of the regulated industry and the FDA staff. This approach has served two purposes. The guidance document can help assure that when a premarket application is submitted to FDA it will contain the data the agency expects for evaluation and determination of the device's clearance or approvability. It also provides a public statement on FDA's policy so everyone in the industry knows what the rules are and everyone, therefore, is treated in an equal and unbiased manner.

It is important to remember that guidance documents are advisory and not binding on the FDA or the manufacturer. This means that FDA may, under certain circumstances, require testing that may differ from or add to the testing called for in a guidance document. The need to assure the effectiveness and safety of the device for patient use is paramount in such situations. Also, if a manufacturer deviates from a guidance document, it must be prepared to justify the deviation and show that its testing method is an adequate substitution for the recommended method.

For examples of the types of nonclinical testing and reports that would be expected for different types of devices, it is instructive to look at some

FDA guidance documents. The following two guidance documents are particularly illustrative of such nonclinical testing:

- "Non-Clinical Information for Femoral Stem Prostheses," which can be found at:

  http://www.fda.gov/MedicalDevices/DeviceRegulationand
  Guidance/GuidanceDocuments/ucm071275.htm

- "Non-Clinical Engineering Tests and Recommended Labeling for Intravascular Stents and Associated Delivery Systems," which can be found at:

  http://www.fda.gov/MedicalDevices/DeviceRegulationand
  Guidance/GuidanceDocuments/ucm071863.htm

It would be wise for a device designer to look into the availability of an applicable FDA guidance before initiating device testing so that valuable time and resources are not wasted by not performing the correct testing for the specific device under design.

Section 5. Animal Experimentation and Evaluation

In addition to testing in the engineering and chemistry labs, it may be necessary to conduct animal studies. This section discusses the scientific and technical aspects of animal testing to develop the data that may be required by FDA. The regulations applicable to animal testing are discussed below in part 2, Good Laboratory Practices.

Animal Model

In animal testing, it is important that an appropriate animal model be chosen for the device and its intended use. The animal model itself, as well as the anatomical site for the use of the device, can affect the outcome of the testing and the device's relationship to human use. The skeletal maturity of the animal may be of concern for certain types of devices, such as orthopedic devices.

Testing and Reporting Factors

The purpose of animal testing on a medical device is to gather data and information for submission to FDA for review and evaluation. In determining the parameters of testing for this use, there are many factors that have to be taken into account, and the details of all animal studies should be clearly specified. Below are some considerations that are important in designing and conducting appropriate testing. They are also important because they will have to be included in the submission to FDA.

The purpose of the testing has to be clearly defined. The test definition should include the control used and explain how the testing will produce the necessary functional and safety evaluations of the device.

Another early consideration is whether the testing should be conducted using the final device or whether component testing is sufficient. Components should be used only if the test results can be translated to the device in its final form.

The methods used for the processing and fixation of histological evaluation must be employed in a manner that does not distort the results that will be used in an application to FDA. The necessary pathological or histological data and information must be identified, as well as how and when they were gathered and presented:

- If radiological data and information are required, the choice of imaging techniques (X-ray, MRI, and CT scan) will have to be determined and justified.

- The instrumentation used in conducting the tests can be important. If the instrumentation is intended for animal use only, it may not produce results that are applicable to the human model.

- When surrogate end points are used, they must be validated. A rationale should be included to explain any differences between the use of the product in animal studies and its intended use in a clinical study.

- Studies should be performed by competent individuals and laboratories following good laboratory practices (GLPs), as discussed in part 2 below.

Duration of Studies

Issues may arise in the conduct of animal studies related to the duration of the study. How long a test article has to be followed depends on the device and its intended use. For example, for an orthopedic fracture fixation device FDA recommends 12 months of test data. Other devices may require shorter or longer periods of follow-up. The species, animal size, and degradation properties of the device can influence the duration of the study. The duration may also be affected by the maturity or development of the animal species.

Section 6. Biocompatibility

Depending on the composition of the device, animal studies may be necessary to establish the biocompatibility of the device if it will come into contact with the human body. This is a particular issue for polymeric ingredients, degradable components, animal-sourced substances, and novel materials. It may also depend on how the manufacturing process might affect the biocompatibility of the device. This type of testing should reveal any potential for adverse events or allergic reactions, and may be used to establish preliminary levels of toxicity.

The biocompatibility tests should be selected to match the patient exposure to the device. Standards are very helpful in this regard. Two major standards that contain guidance on biocompatibility testing are:

- *ISO 10993 Biological evaluation of medical devices*

- *ASTM F748-06 Standard Practice for Selecting Generic Biological Test Methods for Materials and Devices*

FDA also has a guidance document on biocompatibility testing, which provides general guidance on such testing and, in addition, harmonizes the FDA requirements with the biocompatibility testing required by other countries. This guidance is part of Blue Book Memorandum #G95-1 and is entitled "Use of International Standard ISO-10993, 'Biological Evaluation of Medical Devices Part 1: Evaluation and Testing.'" The guidance can be found at:

> http://www.fda.gov/MedicalDevices/DeviceRegulationand
> Guidance/GuidanceDocuments/ucm080735.htm

This guidance contains the following useful attachments that are recommended to those conducting biocompatibility testing of a medical device:

- Attachment A:

    Table 1 Initial Evaluation Tests for Consideration

- Attachment B:

    Table 2 Supplementary Evaluation Tests for Consideration

- Attachment C:

    Biocompatibility Flow Chart for the Selection of Toxicity Tests for 510(k)s (Appears at the end of the guidance)

In designing the biocompatibility testing, an assessment of all available information, including nonclinical, clinical, and post-market information, should be considered, and testing should be completed on a final, processed, sterilized device to demonstrate biocompatibility. Biocompatibility testing should be reconsidered whenever changes are made in the device's composition, processing, configuration, or intended use.

Section 7. Sterility and Shelf Life

Sterility

Another type of nonclinical testing is sterility testing. This is critical if the device is intended for sterile use or the device is intended for use in sterilizing other products. The sterilization method, such as steam, ethylene oxide, gamma radiation, and so on, will be important in determining the test method and validation point. The testing should provide results for the sterility assurance level (SAL) or ethylene oxide residuals (in mg/day).

Manufacturers of medical devices must validate processes, including sterilization, for a device purporting to be sterile. Stability testing should be part of the design validation of such devices. When a product is labeled as sterile, it is considered to be a stability characteristic and must be tested for shelf life, as discussed below.

The sterility testing should take into account the mechanical performance of the device, the integrity of the packaging, the shipping and transportation methods, and any other environmental factors that could affect the sterility of the device up to the time of use.

FDA has a guidance document entitled "Container and Closure System Integrity Testing in Lieu of Sterility Testing As a Component of the Stability Protocol for Sterile Products." It sets forth considerations for demonstrating the continued sterility of products based on the container and closure system used for the product. This guidance was developed jointly by three FDA Centers and deals with FDA-regulated device, drug, and biological products. It also provides citations to other non-FDA guidances on sterility of medical products. The guidance can be found at:

http://www.fda.gov/RegulatoryInformation/Guidances/ucm 146074.htm

If the device is intended for sterile use but not supplied in a sterile condition, the product's labeling must provide appropriate sterilization and validation instructions.

Stability/Shelf Life

The purpose of stability testing is to provide evidence on how the quality of a substance or product varies with time under the influence of a variety of environmental factors such as temperature, humidity, and light. Such testing enables the manufacturer to establish or modify recommended storage conditions, retest periods, and shelf life or dating period, as the case may be.

Shelf life testing is important for products subject to degradation over time. In addition to the factors mentioned above, the length of shelf life may, especially for long-term implantable devices, depend on the specific bodily fluids with which the device may come into contact.

Whether it is possible to use accelerated testing will depend on the materials involved. Where the device includes resorbable polymeric materials, shelf life should be adequately supported and substantiated by real-time testing.

PART 2. GOOD LABORATORY PRACTICE

Nonclinical laboratory testing is governed by FDA's Good Laboratory Practice (GLP) regulation. The primary purpose of this regulation is to assure the quality and integrity of the data, especially safety data.

Section 1. Scope and Applicability

Scope of the Regulation

The GLP regulation applies to all nonclinical laboratory studies that support or are intended to support "applications for research or marketing permits" for products regulated by the FDA.

It covers *in vitro* or *in vivo* experiments on a "test article" in a "test system." The test article may be a drug, device, food substance, biologic, or animal drug. The test system is defined as any animal, plant, microorganism, or their subparts, to which the test or control article is administered or added for study.

Thus, if the nonclinical laboratory testing does not involve a test system as defined, the GLP regulation would not be applicable, but they would, nevertheless, be instructive on the topic of good laboratory practices because they contain many principles and procedures unrelated to the official test systems that should be considered for application in any laboratory environment.

A laboratory that conducts testing in compliance with the GLPs is considered to be a "GLP lab." Laboratories that do not claim to be GLP compliant may or may not be able to conduct studies in compliance with this regulation. If a study is supposed to be conducted in accordance with GLPs, it is important to make sure a capable and competent lab is engaged, or the time and expense of the study may be wasted.

Testing Issues

GLPs do not apply to exploratory studies or basic research designed to evaluate physical characteristics or chemical characteristics. Similarly, the

GLPs do not apply to studies utilizing human subjects in a clinical trial, consumer usability testing, or consumer preference testing.

Section 2. The GLP Regulatory Scheme

The GLP regulation covers the following topics that are discussed in this chapter:

- Organization and personnel
- Facilities
- Equipment
- Testing facilities operations
- Test and control articles
- Protocols
- Records and reports
- Disqualification of testing facilities

Section 3. Organization and Personnel

Personnel

Personnel in a GLP lab must have the education, training, and experience needed to conduct the assigned activities. The facility must maintain records of employees' training, experience, and their job descriptions, and there must be a sufficient number of personnel to perform all of the required duties.

The lab must maintain sanitary conditions and health precautions to avoid contamination of test and control articles and test systems. Personnel must be appropriately clothed to prevent microbiological, radiological, or chemical contamination during testing. Ill individuals that may adversely affect the quality and integrity of the testing must be excluded from the testing.

Study Director

The lab must have a director who is a scientist or other professional of appropriate education, training, and experience. The director has responsibility for the technical conduct of the study and its interpretation, analysis, documentation, and reporting, and must assure that:

- The protocol, discussed in section 8 below, is approved, including changes, and that the protocol is followed.

- All data, including unanticipated responses, are accurately recorded and reported.

- Unforeseen circumstances that may affect the quality and integrity of the study are noted, corrected, and documented.

- GLP regulations are followed.

- All raw data, documentation, protocols, specimens, and final reports are archived.

Quality Assurance Unit

The GLPs require that the lab has a quality assurance unit (QAU) that is entirely separate from and independent of the study personnel. This unit is responsible for monitoring each study to assure management that the facility, equipment, personnel, methods, practices, records, and controls are in compliance with regulatory requirements.

Section 4. Facilities

In general, the laboratory facilities must be of a suitable size and construction to assure a degree of separation to prevent untoward effects on the study. The facility has to be an appropriate laboratory suitable for carrying out the type of studies that will be conducted there, for example, engineering lab, chemistry lab, micro lab.

Facilities for Animal Care

When animals are used as test systems, the lab must have a sufficient number of animal rooms or areas to assure proper:

- Separation of species and test systems

- Isolation of individual projects

- Quarantine of animals

- Routine or specialized housing of animals

- Separation of diseased animals

In addition, there must be separate rooms or areas to ensure isolation of biohazardous materials such as volatile substances, aerosols, radioactive materials, and infectious agents.

General animal care needs must be met, so the lab will require appropriate facilities for the sanitary collection and disposal of animal waste refuse and prevention of vermin infestation, odors, disease hazards, and environmental contamination. There should be separate supply facilities for feed, bedding, equipment, and test systems, which are protected from contamination or infestation, and there should be separate areas for the following:

- Receipt and storage of test and control articles
- Mixing test and control articles
- Storage of test and control article mixtures
- Separation of test and control articles from test and control mixtures
- Operating areas for procedures
- Specimen and data storage, limited to authorized personnel

Section 5. Equipment

Equipment must be inspected, cleaned, tested, calibrated, and standardized. SOPs must specify the methods, materials, and schedules for routine inspection, cleaning, maintenance, testing, calibration, and standardization of equipment. Also, records of the foregoing routine and nonroutine activities must be maintained, including any specifics concerning the discovery and repair of defects.

Section 6. Testing Facilities Operations

Written standard operating procedures are required to assure the quality and integrity of the study data. The SOPs must be established for: animal room preparation; animal care; receipt, identification, storage, handling, and sampling of test and control articles; test system observation; lab tests; handling of dead animals; post-mortems; collection and identification of specimens; histopathology; data handling, storage, and retrieval; maintenance and calibration of equipment; and transfer, placement, and identification of animals. Such manuals and SOPs must be available in each lab area. The lab must maintain a historical file of SOP adoptions, revisions, and dates.

Reagents and solutions must be labeled with identity, titer, storage requirements, and expiration dates.

The GLP regulation enumerates specific animal care requirements:

- SOPs must be established for housing, feeding, handling, and care of animals.

- Newly received animals must be isolated and evaluated in accordance with acceptable veterinary medical practice.

- Sick animals may be treated and used if the illness or treatment does not interfere with the testing.

- Each animal must be identifiable, and identification shall appear on the outside of the unit.

- Animal storage units must be cleaned and sanitized at appropriate intervals.

- Food and water must be analyzed for contaminants that may interfere with the testing, and the results of the analyses recorded.

- Bedding must not interfere with the testing and must be dry and clean.

- Only noninterfering pest control materials may be used and must be documented.

Section 7. Test and Control Articles

Special requirements apply to test and control articles, including the following:

- The identification, strength, purity, and composition of home-brew test and control articles must be defined. For commercial products, the label will characterize them.

- Stability must be tested before or during the testing in accordance with written SOPs.

- The label must contain the name, chemical abstract or code number, expiration date, and storage conditions.

- For studies lasting more than four weeks, reserve test and control articles must be retained in accordance with the record retention rules below.

Section 8. Protocols

Protocol for a Nonclinical Study

Each study must have an approved written protocol that includes:

- A descriptive title and objective of the study

- The identification of the test and control articles

- The name of the sponsor and the name and address of the test facility

- The experimental design, including methods for the control of bias

- The type and frequency of tests, analysis, and measurements to be made

- An identification of the records to be maintained

- The date and approval of the sponsor and the study director

If animals are used, in addition to the foregoing, there must be information concerning:

- The number, body weight, sex, source, species, strain, sub-strain, and age of animals

- Detailed dietary information

- Dosage levels, and route and frequency of administration

Protocol Conformance

A study and the monitoring of the study must conform to the protocol. Data, other than in automated data collection systems, must be recorded directly, promptly, and legibly in ink, and dated and signed by the person entering the data. Manual or automated data corrections must not obscure the original data, and must be initialed and dated with the reason for the change.

Section 9. Records and Reports

It is important that the necessary records and reports be maintained, as these will be subject to a request from FDA or subject to inspection by FDA.

Reporting Requirements

A final report of each nonclinical lab study must be prepared, and it must include:

- The name and address of the test facility, and the beginning and ending dates

- The objectives and procedures from the protocol

- Identification and characteristics of test and control articles

- The statistical methods used in analysis
- The stability of the test and control articles
- The methods used
- Description of the test system used
- Description of all circumstances that may have adversely affected the quality or integrity of the data
- The names of the study director and all supervisory personnel
- A statement of the transformations, calculations, and operations performed on the data, its analysis, and the conclusions drawn
- Signed and dated reports of each scientist or other professional personnel involved
- The location where all specimens, raw data, and the final report are stored
- The statement prepared and signed by the QAU
- Corrections to the final report must be in the form of an amendment by the study director

In addition to the foregoing, for animal studies the report must contain:

- The number of animals and their sex, weight, source, species, strain, sub-strain, age, and method of identification
- A description of the dosage, regimen, route of administration, and duration

Storage and Retrieval of Records

Records are kept in archives designed for the orderly storage and retrieval of all raw data, documentation, protocols, specimens, and interim and final reports. Records may be kept elsewhere, if documented in the archive, and the archiving function may be contracted out to a third party. Only authorized personnel may enter the archives.

Record Retention

GLP record retention requirements do not replace or supersede other record retention requirements in the regulations. Records, raw data, and specimens must be retained for the lesser of:

- Two years after FDA approval

- Five years after they are submitted to FDA

- Two years after the study is completed, terminated, or discontinued, if the data were not submitted to FDA

Section 10. Disqualification of Testing Facilities

As in the case of a clinical investigator or an IRB, a testing lab may be disqualified by FDA. Disqualification is discussed in Chapter 8, part 2, Compliance Actions and Penalties.

PART 3. EXERCISES

1. Provide a list of the types of testing that might be conducted during the nonclinical testing phase of development of a medical device.

2. What device studies are covered by the Good Laboratory Practice regulation?

3. What studies are not covered by the Good Laboratory Practice regulation?

4. When is a standard operating procedure required, and what is the purpose of an SOP?

5. The president of the company you work for informs you that the board of directors has given the go-ahead for your proposed new soft contact lens. The next step involves the preparation of a procedure for the nonclinical testing of the prototype contact lens. Please draft a nonclinical testing SOP for a specific characteristic of the lens for presentation to the R&D Oversight Committee.

6. The president of the company informed you that the board of directors liked your design plan for the new examination glove and is ready to approve the development, but it needs to know the costs involved. Accordingly, the president has asked the accounting department to work up a cost analysis for the development project. The accounting department has informed the president that it can not do so until it has more-detailed information on all of the steps that have to be taken in the development process. Hence, the president is asking the R&D Oversight Committee to prepare a list of the specific SOPs or protocols necessary for the nonclinical

and clinical testing of the gloves. The committee has assigned to your engineering team the project of preparing the listing of the necessary SOPs and protocols for use by accounting. Please prepare an inventory of the nonclinical tests and the associated SOPs and/or protocols for presentation to the R&D Oversight Committee.

4
Clinical Trials

Experimenting on human beings with an investigational device, even under an authorized clinical trial, raises moral issues, and issues of patient rights, patient safety, and the privacy of the medical condition of the subjects in the trial, along with concerns over the confidentiality and freedom from bias of the data generated by the trial. It is not surprising that the conduct of a clinical trial is heavily regulated by a complex and detailed set of rules and regulations.

Volumes have been written about clinical trials. There are textbooks and articles written on any of these topics that provide a great deal of detailed information about them. This chapter presents an overview of a selection of topics relevant to the design and conduct of clinical trials. Some of the topics covered include clinical trial design, informed consent, institutional review boards, investigational device exemptions, bioresearch monitoring, financial interests of investigators, and registration of clinical trials in a national database.

GOOD CLINICAL PRACTICES

The various rules, principles, and standards governing clinical trials are commonly referred to as *good clinical practices,* or GCPs. Good clinical practice (GCP) is expressed in and represented by a collection of international ethical and scientific quality standards for designing, conducting, recording, and reporting trials that involve human subjects. Compliance with GCP assures that the rights, safety, and well-being of trial subjects are protected and that the clinical trial data are reliable and credible.

Biostatistics

One important topic is not included here because it is specialized and beyond the scope of this book. This is the subject of *biostatistics,* which is very important, if not critical, to the proper design and evaluation of a clinical trial. There are many statistical models that can be considered concerning the number of patients in the study, the construction of patient cohorts, the power and confidence ranges that will be achieved, and so on. Biostatistics textbooks, articles, and other references should be consulted for information on the use and application of the principles of biostatistics.

PART 1. BACKGROUND INFORMATION

Section 1. Regulatory Scheme

In the United States, good clinical practices are embodied in a number of regulations that govern the conduct of clinical trials. The major ones are listed below. All of them have been promulgated by agencies within the Department of Health and Human Services (DHHS), including the FDA and the National Institutes of Health. All of them are enforced by the FDA in regard to the products regulated by FDA and are discussed further in this chapter. The websites where these regulations can be found follow each regulation.

- 21 CFR Part 50, Protection of Human Subjects, provides the requirements and general elements of informed consent.

  http://www.accessdata.fda.gov/scripts/cdrh/cfdocs/cfcfr/
  CFRSearch.cfm?CFRPart=50&showFR=1

- 21 CFR Part 54, Financial Disclosure by Clinical Investigators, covers the disclosure of financial compensation to clinical investigators, which is part of FDA's assessment of the reliability of the clinical data.

  http://www.accessdata.fda.gov/scripts/cdrh/cfdocs/cfcfr/
  CFRSearch.cfm?CFRPart=54&showFR=1

- 21 CFR Part 56, Institutional Review Boards, covers the procedures and responsibilities for institutional review boards (IRBs) that approve and monitor clinical investigations.

  http://www.accessdata.fda.gov/scripts/cdrh/cfdocs/cfcfr/
  CFRSearch.cfm?CFRPart=56&showFR=1

- 21 CFR Part 812, Investigational Device Exemptions, covers the procedures for the conduct of clinical studies with medical devices, including applications, responsibilities of sponsors and investigators, labeling, records, and reports.

  http://www.accessdata.fda.gov/scripts/cdrh/cfdocs/cfcfr/CFRSearch.cfm?CFRPart=812&showFR=1

- 21 CFR Part 820 Subpart C, Design Controls of the Quality System Regulation, provides the requirement for procedures to control the design of the device in order to ensure that the specified design requirements are met.

  http://www.accessdata.fda.gov/scripts/cdrh/cfdocs/cfcfr/CFRSearch.cfm?CFRPart=820&showFR=1

- 21 CFR Part 11, Electronic Records; Electronic Signatures, assures that electronic records maintained in a clinical trial, as well as all other records for FDA-related matters, are trustworthy, reliable, and generally equivalent to paper records and handwritten signatures.

  http://www.accessdata.fda.gov/scripts/cdrh/cfdocs/cfCFR/CFRSearch.cfm?CFRPart=11

- NIH Fact Sheet entitled "Registration at ClinicalTrials.gov: As Required by Public Law 110-85, Title VIII" explains the registration system for clinical trials in the clinicaltrials.gov database.

  http://prsinfo.clinicaltrials.gov/s801-fact-sheet.pdf

Section 2. International Guidelines for Medical Device Research

The international community has developed various rules and guidelines for the regulation of medical research. These are important because, according to FDA, approximately 20 percent of the clinical studies submitted in support of a PMA application are conducted outside the United States. Each foreign study should be performed in accordance with the Declaration of Helsinki or the laws and regulations of the country in which the study is conducted. If the study is conducted in accordance with the laws of the country, the PMA applicant is required to explain to FDA in detail the differences between the laws of the country and the Declaration of Helsinki.

The major international compilations of international guidelines are described on the CODEX Web site and can be found at the link appearing after the following CODEX quotation:

Together with the Helsinki Declaration, "Good Clinical Practice" and "International Ethical Guidelines for Biomedical Research Involving Human Subjects" are the most important and most used international rule compilations for medical research. Together with WHO, The Council for International Organizations of Medical Sciences" (CIOMS) has issued International Ethical Guidelines for Biomedical Research Involving Human Subjects (first issued in the '80s), focused on questions concerning security and informed consent. The document attempts to implement the Helsinki Declaration's principles while considering important differences between the world's countries. It includes special provisions on research involving vulnerable groups or women. Then, at the 1996 "International Conference on Harmonization of Technical Requirements for Registration of Pharmaceuticals for Human Use" (ICH), a more technical and specific set of guidelines was created, going under the name "Good Clinical Practice." This document addresses virtually all aspects of experimental work, with special focus on the procedure for application to ethics committees. It is applicable in the U.S. and Japan as well as in the EU. To help European research ethics committees, the "European Forum for Good Clinical Practice" has produced guidelines and recommendations for GCP. Good Clinical Practice can be found in a somewhat different form from WHO—these guidelines' use is more dependent on which country they are to be used in, and they affiliate themselves explicitly with the Helsinki Declaration and CIOMS guidelines, whereas ICH's GCP does not. WHO has also issued a complementary "Handbook for Good Clinical Research Practice."

The EU has issued Directive 2001/20/EC of the European Parliament and of the Council of 4 April 2001 on the approximation of the laws, regulations, and administrative provisions of the Member States relating to the implementation of good clinical practice in the conduct of clinical trials on medicinal products for human use. This was followed by Commission Directive 2005/28/EC laying down principles and detailed guidelines for good clinical practice as regards investigational medicinal products for human use, as well as the requirements for authorization of the manufacturing or importation of such products. According to this directive, all clinical trials shall be "guided by ethical principles in all their aspects." ICH's regulations concerning security, efficiency, and inspection can be found here and EMEA's collection of documents here. The EU regulations are collected in "The Rules Governing Medicinal Products in the European Union."

http://www.codex.vr.se/en/forskningmedicin.shtml

Section 3. Major Clinical Trial Participants and Definitions

The following list identifies and defines some of the major participants in a clinical trial that are identified in one or more of the foregoing regulations. These are the primary actors in the conduct of a clinical trial. They are defined in the definitions section of the regulations, but the definitions of each may differ slightly depending on the regulation in which the definition appears, and its purpose. They all are directly regulated by FDA. There are many professionals and support staff who contribute to the success of a clinical trial, but their activities, although very important, are fulfilling a supportive role. They will be discussed elsewhere in this chapter as the need arises.

- *Sponsor:* "Sponsor" means a person who initiates a clinical investigation but does not necessarily conduct the investigation. This may include an individual practitioner, a device manufacturer, a device designer, an institution, or other organization.

- *Clinical investigator* (CI): "Investigator" means an individual who actually conducts a clinical investigation. This is the physician, dentist, surgeon, or other practitioner who actually administers the device to the subjects in the trial and evaluates the subjects' response to the device.

- *Human subject* (subject): "Human subject" means an individual, including an individual's specimen, who participates in research either as the recipient of a "test article" or as a control. A subject may be in normal health or may have a medical condition or disease.

- *Test article:* "Test article" means any medical device for human use, an investigational device, or any other article subject to regulation under the act.

- *Investigational device:* "Investigational device" means a device, including a transitional device, that is the object of an investigation.

- *Monitor:* "Monitor," when used as a noun, means an individual designated by a sponsor or contract research organization to oversee the progress of an investigation. The monitor may be an employee of a sponsor or a consultant to the sponsor, or an employee of or consultant to a contract research organization. "Monitor," when used as a verb, means to oversee an investigation.

*   *Institution:* "Institution," or "facility," means any public or private entity or agency. As well as hospitals and other healthcare institutions, it includes federal, state, or local agencies such as the NIH, the CDC, the Veterans Administration, the Department of Defense, or state hospitals.

*   *Institutional review board* (IRB): "Institutional review board" means any group designated by an institution to review, approve, or oversee biomedical research involving human subjects.

*   *Contract research organization* (CRO): "Contract research organization" means a person that assumes, as an independent contractor with the sponsor, one or more of the obligations of a sponsor, for example, design of a protocol, selection and monitoring of investigational sites, evaluation of reports, and preparation of materials to be submitted to the Food and Drug Administration.

Other specific definitions are provided elsewhere, as needed.

Section 4. Ethics in Clinical Trials

The National Institutes of Health sponsors and conducts a large number of clinical trials. NIH has invested a great effort in assuring that clinical research is conducted in an ethical manner.

The NIH web page, "Ethics in Clinical Research," lists the following elements that must be considered in determining whether the conduct of a clinical trial meets ethical standards:

*   Social and clinical value

*   Scientific validity

*   Fair subject selection

*   Favorable risk–benefit ratio

*   Independent review

*   Informed consent

*   Respect for potential and enrolled subjects

These topics, and others, are discussed in more detail at:

http://clinicalresearch.nih.gov/ethics_guides.html

The NIH website also discusses various ethical guidelines and, in addition, presents an excellent slide presentation entitled "What Makes Clinical Research Ethical?" which is available online at:

http://www.bioethics.nih.gov/slides/10-29-03-Emmanuel.pdf

Section 5. Bias and Financial Conflicts of Interest

Just as for any other scientific research, all clinical studies have to be objective and free of bias. One of the major sources of bias in a clinical trial can be the financial interest of a clinical investigator. Financial interests can take many forms. It might be a significant equity interest such as stock ownership or other proprietary interest in the company sponsoring the study. It might be an equity interest in a different company that will manufacture and market the device. The financial interest could involve certain types of compensation such as future payments based on the success of the product. It might also include salary or other payments for services (for example, consulting fees or honoraria), and intellectual property rights (for example, patents, copyrights, and royalties from such rights).

Significant financial interests, whatever their nature, may result in the investigator making significant sums of money if the product is a success. This in turn can create a conflict because the clinical investigator holding the interest may be influenced or biased in his or her judgment when evaluating the product being tested.

This issue has attracted a great deal of attention from private patient-interest groups, the National Academy of Sciences' Institute of Medicine, medical journals, the U.S. Congress, and private sector research institutions themselves. They have recommended full reporting and disclosure of such interests so the research results of the investigator may be judged independently by others not so conflicted.

As a major funder of biomedical research, including medical devices, NIH is particularly concerned about the financial interests of those receiving federal funding for this type of research. To deal with this concern, NIH proposed amendments to its regulations in 21 CFR Part 50, Grants and Agreements, and Part 94, Responsible Prospective Contractors, to tighten up the control over financial interests of investigators receiving funding from NIH, including their spouses and dependent children. This proposal and its preamble provide a detailed discussion of the extent of federal funding for biomedical research and the concerns and issues presented by significant financial interests on the part of researchers. Because this regulation is so far-reaching, it will also affect private funding of biomedical research. The proposal can be found at:

http://www.gpo.gov/fdsys/pkg/FR-2010-05-21/pdf/2010-11885.pdf

Some of the more prominent changes that will be brought about by this proposal, if adopted in its current form, include:

- The threshold for reporting financial interests will be reduced from $10,000 to $5000.

- The responsibility for deciding whether a particular relationship is a potential financial conflict of interest will now rest on the institution as opposed to the investigator.

- The institution receiving funding will be required to set up a process to review potential conflicts of interest.

- Institutions will be required to identify those researchers that may need an intervention and to report to NIH its actions in that regard.

- Institutions will now be required to develop a publicly accessible website that will display significant financial interests of their faculty and other institutional members in order for the public to have a clear pathway toward identifying what kinds of arrangements have been made so that there is transparency to the process.

Anyone involved in or planning to be involved in government-funded biomedical research should read the full proposal. It will also be important to be aware of the final regulation and its requirements when issued in final form.

Just as NIH is concerned about financial bias in the research it sponsors, FDA is likewise concerned about the integrity of the clinical data it reviews in marketing applications in evaluating the safety and effectiveness of medical devices. For a discussion of how FDA handles this matter in marketing applications, see Chapter 5, part 1, Global Marketing Application Concepts.

Section 6. Monitoring and Auditing a Clinical Trial

All clinical trials must be monitored, and sometimes the trial must be audited. These processes are applicable to many phases in the design, testing, complaint handling, and manufacturing of a medical device. Rather than repeating the discussion of monitoring and auditing in multiple places throughout the book, the topic is treated in its various forms in Chapter 1, part 11, Monitoring and Auditing.

Section 7. Controls for Clinical Trials

Although the intent and purpose of a clinical trial differs from a nonclinical study, they share some of the same types of controls and functions. For example, a nonclinical study that does not use animals or other life-forms requires an SOP whereas a nonclinical study using animals or other life-forms and clinical trials require a protocol. Both the SOP and the protocol serve the same basic purpose in these studies. All nonclinical studies and clinical trials require qualified personnel, adequate facilities, record keeping, reports, and other parallel functions and controls of the same general nature.

However, because of a major difference in a clinical trial, that is, the use of human subjects, the rules for a clinical trial are more elaborate and more specific for the purpose of protecting human subjects and for assuring the quality of the outcomes concerning the ultimate safety and effectiveness (S&E) of the device that may be drawn from generally more complex and sometimes confounding data.

Some clinical trials may present a significant risk (SR) to the subjects in the trial. Other trials may present a nonsignificant risk (NSR). The differences in the regulatory status of SR and NSR studies are discussed below in part 5, Investigational Device Exemptions.

One of the purposes of this chapter is to provide information specific to clinical trials, just as Chapter 3 provided details about nonclinical studies.

PART 2. CLINICAL TRIAL DESIGN

Section 1. The Investigational Plan

An investigational plan and a protocol are critical to the proper conduct of a clinical trial, and essential for obtaining FDA approval of an IDE. IRBs reviewing a proposed clinical trial will expect to see most of these same elements in the plan it reviews. The elements that are expected in an investigational plan include:

- The purpose
- The protocol
- A risk analysis
- A description of the device
- Monitoring procedures

- Labeling

- IRB information

- A report of prior investigations

- Additional records and reports

One important item that sometimes may be overlooked is the requirement to report prior investigations of the investigational device. This report should include a bibliography of publications relevant to an evaluation of the safety or effectiveness of the device, whether that information is adverse or supportive of the device. It should include a summary of all other unpublished information, whether adverse or supportive. For nonclinical laboratory studies, the report should state whether the studies were in compliance with GLPs, and if not in compliance, explain why.

Section 2. The Clinical Trial Protocol

The heart of a clinical trial plan is the clinical trial protocol. The protocol defines all of the aspects of the clinical trial design that must be followed during the trial. The protocol is a document that is reviewed by the IRB for all studies and, in addition, by FDA for IDE studies. The IRB and the FDA will review the protocol in detail before approving a clinical trial. Rarely is a protocol approved without some discussion between the sponsor and FDA, often resulting in some changes, and sometimes ending with significant modifications being required before approval. There are even times when a protocol is so unacceptable it will not be approved and it will have to be completely rewritten.

When approved, the protocol is provided to the clinical investigators to be used and followed in the conduct of the trial. Because of its critical importance, the following sections discuss various elements of the clinical protocol. The protocol is a variable document, with the elements depending on the nature of the device, the procedures to be used, and the purpose of the study.

The Purpose of a Clinical Trial

Clinical trials are used for several purposes. Many clinical trials are used to obtain data for submission to FDA to obtain marketing approval for a medical device. If the application is a Premarket Approval (PMA) application, which is discussed in Chapter 5, part 3, PMAs/PDPs/HDEs, the clinical trial will be used to establish the safety and effectiveness (S&E) of a new device. Another use is to show the S&E of a new use for an approved device in a PMA supplement. There are cases where a study may be conducted to show that a product is superior or not inferior to another product. Sometimes a clinical trial is required to demonstrate substantial equivalence in a premarket notification (510[k]), which is discussed in Chapter 5, part 2, Premarket Notification (510[k]).

Not all clinical trials, however, are conducted to obtain data for marketing approval. Some clinical trials are conducted for basic research purposes to obtain scientific information or to establish a new scientific principle. Other trials may be conducted to try a new technique for the administration of an approved device. Some sponsors/investigators want to develop comparative information for use in their practices. Also, a small clinical trial may be conducted to show the feasibility of using a device in a larger clinical trial.

Planning the Trial

Prospective planning is the key to a successful study. The protocol should be based on sound science and described in a clear and detailed manner. The objectives and the expected outcomes of the trial must be clearly stated. It should identify the hypotheses to be tested. Whatever the goal of the study may be, it needs to be formulated into a statistical study hypothesis. The same basic steps are applicable to a clinical trial as those for nonclinical studies. See Table 3.1 in Chapter 3.

Section 3. Blinding

The protocol should address what type of blinding the study will use. The most desirable study is a double-blind study. In a double-blind study, neither the patient nor the physician knows whether the patient is receiving the investigational device or a placebo. When this blinding is used, it eliminates the risk of bias entering into the evaluation of the product by the patient or the physician. It also clearly exposes any "placebo effect" the device may have. The *placebo effect* is the favorable response and evaluation by the patient or physician based solely on their expectations of a product that is otherwise inert, with no effectiveness.

Because of the nature of medical device research where identifiable devices are used by the investigator, for example, an orthopedic surgeon, a single-blind study is more likely, where the patient is the only one who does not know whether the test device has been implanted. When this is the case, the blinding in the study may occur at the time of evaluation. In other words, the evaluator will be a qualified practitioner who did not perform the surgery and does not know which subjects received the test device. This third-party practitioner will review the outcome during a follow-up exam or by reading postsurgical X-ray images of the subjects.

Not all trials can be blinded. If the product is an obvious implant that can not be masked, there will be no blinding. The surgeon will know that the investigational device is being used, and so will the patient. Another reason a trial may not be blinded is because the patient is seriously ill and has no other treatment options, and the device has an acceptable level of probability that it will work. In life-threatening situations, the decision may be made that it is worth the chance to use the device in an effort to save a patient's life.

Section 4. Study Controls

Concurrent Control

The type of study control that will be used during the trial is an important subject for the protocol. The protocol should explain whether the trial will have a concurrent control or historical control. A *concurrent control* is one in which the investigational device is compared to a sham or placebo device or another marketed device that would be considered the "control."

Historical Control

In *historical controls,* the investigational device is compared to the performance of other devices that have been previously studied and for which test data are available. Data from previous studies may be available in the files of the sponsor, other sponsors, universities and clinics, or in the published literature.

Some sponsors prefer studies with historical controls based on the belief that they are less expensive than one with traditional controls. However, studies with historical controls may be riskier than studies with concurrent controls. The patient populations may not be the same. It is sometimes difficult to find a historical patient population that is similar enough to the study population to yield reliable study results. For example, if FDA finds that the historical population was not as healthy as the study population, it may disqualify the study because the historical reference will make the device look better than it really is. On the other hand, if the patients in the historical control were in better health than the patients in the device study, the device may look worse, even if it is better. Either scenario may be costly for the sponsor and not achieve the desired evaluation by the agency. Having a concurrent control eliminates differences in patient populations as a source of bias.

Fixed Target Value

An alternative type of study without a concurrent control is one in which the test article is compared to a fixed target value. In this case there is generally no other device for comparison, and the study will measure its results against predetermined end points.

Section 5. Number of Patients and Study Sites

The subjects or patients and study sites in the study are also topics for the protocol. The following considerations are some of the factors related to the patients and study sites in planning the clinical trial.

Study Sites

The first question to consider deals with how many centers will carry out the trial. Will there be one center or will the study be multicentered? Multiple centers are generally preferred because it provides an opportunity to compare results obtained at one center with the results obtained at other centers. When this cross-center comparison is analyzed, it may yield results that confirm the consistency of outcomes, which will have greater probative value. On the other hand, it may show a bias in one center compared to another center. If the results at different centers are significantly different, it also may demonstrate a weakness in the protocol or shortcomings in the selection or training of the different clinical investigators. FDA will always examine the consistency of results across all centers in a study.

Determining the number of study sites that are desirable for a study is sometimes related to the number of patients in the study. It would not be unreasonable, as an intuitive matter, to conclude that more patients in a study would require more study sites while fewer patients would require fewer study sites. This, however, is not always true. For example, there have been studies with large patient populations and only a few study sites. Such a study may have required the skill of clinical investigators of which there were only a few available throughout the country. There have also been studies with only a handful of patients at several study sites. It may have been that the study was dealing with a disease or condition that is relatively rare, and it was necessary to have many study sites in order to attract a sufficient number of subjects to produce meaningful results.

Patient Inclusion/Exclusion Criteria

A basic question that has to be answered by the protocol is who will be included as a subject in the study. The inclusion criteria will be used to determine whether a particular individual is suitable for participation in the trial. A most critical factor in patient selection is whether the individual has the disease or condition for which the device is intended. There will most likely be other characteristics that must be met to qualify for participation in the trial, such as age, sex, race, and so on.

The screening for participation in the trial will also look at whether the individual meets some exclusion criterion, and there may be many. Depending on each particular study, some examples of exclusion criteria that might be applied include: women of child bearing age, taking certain medications, having had previous treatments for the disease or condition, and the unavailability of the individual for follow-up examinations. There are many more reasons why an individual may have to be excluded from a clinical trial, and these have to be identified in the clinical protocol and applied by the clinical investigator during the conduct of the trial.

Subject Sample Size and Study Cohorts

The number of patients included in the study is critical to the analysis of the results of the study. Sample size should be calculated from the study hypothesis depending, in part, on how big a treatment effect is expected. FDA will want enough subjects in the study to provide statistical significance. The agency does not want more patients than necessary because it could result in unnecessarily exposing subjects to the risks of an unproven device. This is a decision in which a statistician should be consulted to determine the desirable sample size.

The patients enrolled in a study must then be assigned to a study cohort. Often there will be two study cohorts. One cohort will receive the treatment device, and the other group—the control group—will not. The control group may receive a sham device or an approved device already on the market.

Sometimes there are more than two cohorts. There may be more than one treatment group if more than one effect of the device is to be tested, such as in the case of a combination product. There may be more than one control group also. Each control group may use a different method for comparison. For example, the different groups might receive a sham device, a drug, surgery, or no treatment at all. Then the device can be compared to different treatment modalities.

Once the number of subjects and cohorts has been established, the protocol must specify a method for randomly assigning subjects to each of the cohorts. In a double-blind study, the randomization would be made such that the clinical investigator does not know which subject is in which group. There are computer programs for this use.

Duration of Follow-Up

The purpose of patient follow-up after being treated in a clinical trial is to determine how long the treatment with the device will be effective and to determine whether there are any long-term adverse effects from the use of the device. The length of follow-up depends on the type of device and how long it is intended to last. For example, some implants are intended to last for many years. In these cases a lengthier follow-up would be required.

FDA does not want to keep beneficial technology off the market unnecessarily when it can improve health or save lives. Therefore, evaluations are made after some reasonable period of follow-up. Sometimes, the preclinical testing for long-term durability can be combined with clinical data that assess short- to mid-term outcomes, and the device can be approved for marketing. Other times, the agency may require post-market studies that might go on for years to determine the long-term effect of the device.

Section 6. Proving Safety and Effectiveness and Substantial Equivalence

Most clinical trials are designed to provide reasonable assurances of the safety and effectiveness (S&E) of the test article. When a clinical trial is used for this purpose, a pivotal study must be designed to demonstrate the reasonable assurance of both safety and effectiveness. For this reason, the protocol should include a primary safety end point and a primary effectiveness end point. The FDA will use these data in determining whether the device is safe and effective. This evaluation is made during the review of the PMA, and is discussed in Chapter 5, part 3, PMAs/PDPs/HDEs.

There are also clinical trials that are used to show that a test device is substantially equivalent (SE) to an appropriate predicate device. The use of a clinical trial for this latter purpose is discussed under Chapter 5, part 2, Premarket Notification (510[k]).

In either of these cases, the sample size calculations must address safety and effectiveness or substantial equivalence.

Study End Points

The protocol must identify the primary end points determining safety or effectiveness, or both, depending on the purpose of the study, and it should also identify any secondary end points that are being sought. Sometimes, if the primary end point is not met, an argument can be made for approval based on corroborative information from other studies published in the literature, or based on a modification of the indications for use or the addition of cautions or warnings to the label. Whether this approach will work depends on the intended use of the device and the seriousness of the risks it may present in patient care.

Indications for Use of the Device

FDA approves devices for specific indications. The clinical study should be designed to reflect the intended uses of the device and the intended patient population. It is very important that the protocol indentify these parameters before conducting a pivotal clinical study. The indications for use of the device are critical to the establishment of required end points and evaluation for a determination of S&E or SE. Without knowing what the device is intended for, it is impossible to say whether the device has met the standard for either S&E or SE.

Retrospective Analysis

If the study fails to show safety and effectiveness in the target population, firms may be tempted to conduct retrospective subgroup analyses to identify a patient population that may benefit. For example, when a clinical study does not show effectiveness in all heart failure patients, a retrospective analysis may show some effectiveness in the sickest heart failure patients. Such retrospective analyses are not statistically valid and will generally not be sufficient to support approval. The probability of seeing a positive result that is due strictly to chance increases each time a retrospective subgroup analysis is performed. Analyzing enough subgroups will eventually find one that benefits from the device.

PART 3. INFORMED CONSENT

Section 1. General Applicability

FDA regulates clinical investigations intended to gather information in support of applications for research or marketing permits. This includes data or information supporting IDEs, 510(k)s, PMAs, humanitarian device exemptions (HDEs), product development protocols (PDPs), a classification determination, or a medical device standard. A major responsibility in the regulation of a clinical trial is assuring that the clinical investigator obtains the written, signed, and legally effective informed consent for each subject in the trial prior to the administration of the investigational device or the control. An investigator must obtain the informed consent from the human subject or the subject's legally authorized representative.

Section 2. IRB and FDA Review and Approval of Informed Consent Form

The informed consent form will be submitted as part of the investigational plan submitted to an IRB or, in the case of an IDE, submitted additionally to FDA. These organizations will review the informed consent form and, if necessary, request or require modification of the form so that the subject is fully informed at the time of consenting to participation in the trial and signing the form.

Section 3. Elements of Informed Consent

An acceptable informed consent must provide adequate and full disclosure, there must be no coercion or undue influence involved in obtaining the consent, and the consent form may not contain any exculpatory language. *Exculpatory language* is language that would have the subject waive some legal recourse the subject might subsequently pursue against the investigator or sponsor should a serious unexpected event occur due to the fault of the sponsor or investigator. Such events may include negligence, misrepresentation, or other conduct that causes harm to the patient and for which the patient may have legal recourse in a court of law.

An effective informed consent must cover and explain each of the following points in the written consent form:

- The purpose, length of time, and procedures

- Any foreseeable risks and discomforts

- The reasonably expected benefits

- Any available alternative procedures or treatments

- The confidentiality of records

- The possibility of FDA inspection of records

- The availability of compensation and available treatments for injuries

- Identification of contacts for research information, subjects' rights, and research-related injuries

- That participation is voluntary and may be discontinued at any time without loss of benefits

- The following statement:

  "A description of this clinical trial will be available on http://www.clinicaltrials.gov, as required by U.S. law. This website will not include information that can identify you. At most, the website will include a summary of the results. You can search this website at any time."

Additional topics that may also require discussion in the consent form include:

- Whether there may be unforeseen risks to the subject or fetus

- Circumstances under which participation may be discontinued without subject consent

- Consequences if subject withdraws from the study

- That new findings and information arising during the study affecting the subject's participation will be provided

- The additional costs to the subject

- The approximate number of subjects in the study

Section 4. Documentation of Informed Consent

The clinical site must provide a copy of the full written consent form, signed by the subject or his or her representative, to the signer. Alternatively, the site may provide a short written consent form and must present all of the elements of the full consent form verbally in the presence of a witness, provided the IRB approves the written summary and what will be said. The subject must sign the full consent form, and the witness must sign both the consent form and the summary.

Section 5. Emergency Use Exception from Informed Consent

There may be times when an emergency situation arises in which the traditional informed consent can not be obtained before an investigational device is administered. The regulations allow this treatment if the following conditions are met:

1. The site obtains a certification in writing by the investigator and a physician not connected to the study that all of the following apply:

   a. It is a life-threatening situation requiring the use of the test article.

   b. The subject is unable to communicate or grant an effective informed consent.

   c. There is insufficient time to get consent from a legal representative.

   d. No alternative approved or generally recognized therapy with equal or greater likelihood of saving the subject's life is available.

2. If the emergency does not allow time to obtain a second opinion per item 1 above, then after using the test article, the investigator must obtain the written review and evaluation of a physician not connected to the study within five (5) working days after the use of the article.

3. The documentation required in 1 or 2 above must be submitted to the IRB within five (5) working days after the use of the test article.

Section 6. Special Safeguards for Children

An IRB may approve a clinical trial involving children only if:

- It is of minimal risk, and the IRB documents adequate provisions for soliciting the assent of the children and the permission of the parents.

- It is of greater than minimal risk but holds out the prospect of direct benefit to the individual subject, or there is a monitoring procedure that is likely to contribute to the subject's well-being, and both of the following apply:
  – The risk is justified by the anticipated benefit.
  – The benefit is at least as great as that of alternative treatments.

- It is of greater than minimal risk without an anticipated benefit to the individual, but it is likely to yield generalized knowledge about the subject's disorder or condition or present an opportunity to understand, alleviate, or prevent a serious problem affecting children.

Section 7. In Vitro Diagnostic Device (IVD) Testing

Under current regulations, a *human subject* includes an individual on whose specimens an investigational device is used. Because these regulations require informed consent for FDA-regulated human subject research, except in limited circumstances specified in the regulations, informed consent is required before specimens can be used in FDA-regulated research.

Enforcement Exception for Certain IVDs

Due to the difficulty of obtaining informed consent for the use of some specimens, FDA has issued a guidance document that deals with this problem entitled "Informed Consent for In Vitro Diagnostic Device Studies

Using Leftover Human Specimens That Are Not Individually Identifiable."
This guidance can be found at:

> http://www.fda.gov/MedicalDevices/DeviceRegulationand
> Guidance/GuidanceDocuments/ucm078384.htm

Under this guidance:

> FDA does not intend to object to the use, without informed consent,
> of leftover human specimens—remnants of specimens collected
> for routine clinical care or analysis that would otherwise have been
> discarded—in investigations that meet the criteria for exemption
> from the Investigational Device Exemptions (IDE) regulation at
> 21 CFR 812.2(c)(3), as long as subject privacy is protected by
> using only specimens that are not individually identifiable. FDA
> also intends to include in this policy specimens obtained from
> specimen repositories and specimens that are left over from speci-
> mens previously collected for other unrelated research, as long as
> these specimens are not individually identifiable.

Potential Terrorism Exception for IVDs

In clinical trials for the testing of in vitro diagnostic devices, it is necessary to obtain the informed consent of the individual from whom the blood,
urine, or tissue sample is derived. However, in the case of an investigational
in vitro diagnostic device used to identify chemical, biological, radiological, or nuclear agents, the requirement to obtain informed consent is waived
if the patient's life is at risk, if time and conditions do not permit obtaining
the informed consent of the patient or his or her representative, and there is
no cleared or approved method of diagnosis available.

PART 4. INSTITUTIONAL
REVIEW BOARDS

An institutional review board (IRB) is a special committee that has regulatory responsibility for clinical trials regulated by FDA. An IRB is usually associated with a healthcare institution such as a hospital. An IRB also
may be created by a private organization that offers IRB services to sponsors and investigators conducting clinical trials. In either case, the primary
purpose of an IRB is to assure the protection of the rights and welfare of
humans who become subjects in a clinical trial. In doing so, the IRB has
many responsibilities and duties as discussed below.

Section 1. IRB Structure and Membership

The regulations require that an IRB be structured to represent a combination of skill sets so that various aspects of the clinical trial receive adequate consideration. It can not consist of all scientists or all medical personnel. In this manner, other interests of the subject's well-being and welfare, as well as ethical factors, can be addressed, as opposed to addressing just the scientific needs of the trial.

To meet this goal, the regulations require that an IRB consist of at least five members who, as a group, are (1) professionally competent to review the studies, (2) diverse in experience, expertise, gender, and race, (3) knowledgeable in applicable standards and professional conduct, (4) knowledgeable in applicable laws, regulations, and institutional policies, and (5) sensitive to safeguarding the rights and welfare of human subjects.

In addition to the foregoing, the IRB may not consist of all men or all women. There must be at least one member whose primary concern is with scientific matters. There must be one member whose primary concerns are in nonscientific areas, such as an ethicist, clergyman, lawyer, patient rights advocate, and so on. One of the members must be unaffiliated with the sponsoring institution, and no member may have a conflicting interest in the study under review, such as a financial interest in the investigational device. The IRB is always free to invite specialists to consult on specific projects.

Section 2. IRB Duties and Responsibilities

The IRB has responsibilities in connection with all medical device clinical trials subject to FDA's investigational device exemption (IDE) regulation. The IDE regulation is discussed below in part 5, Investigational Device Exemptions. The IRB provides oversight for significant risk studies, which require approval by FDA, and nonsignificant risk studies that do not require FDA approval. The IRB does not provide oversight for nonclinical laboratory studies. It may also have other duties concerning patient care within the institution unrelated to the use of investigational studies, but these other duties are not within the scope of this book.

Specific Functions and Duties

In its capacity as overseer of a clinical trial, an IRB has certain designated functions it must carry out, including the following:

- Review of research

- Approval of research

- Review of informed consent documents and records

- Periodic reviews

- Review by the institution

- Suspension or termination of approved research

- Cooperative research

- Monitoring the research

The seminal act of the IRB is to approve clinical trials. In doing so, the IRB must take into account various factors and make certain determinations before approving a clinical trial. The IRB must make sure the risks to subjects in the trial are minimized and that the risks to subjects are reasonable in relation to the anticipated benefits. It must also assure that the selection of subjects is equitable. It must pay particular attention to vulnerable populations, for example, children, prisoners, pregnant women, the handicapped, or mentally disabled persons.

The IRB must be sure the sponsor and clinical investigators are performing their necessary duties. The IRB must assure that they are in compliance with informed consent requirements and that there is adequate monitoring. The IRB must also make sure patient privacy is protected.

Records and Reports

The IRB must maintain a variety of records related to the trials it has under its jurisdiction, including the following:

- Copies of all research proposals, evaluations, sample consent documents, progress reports, and reports of injuries

- Minutes of IRB meetings (attendance, actions and their rationale, votes, summary of discussion of controversial issues/ resolution)

- Records of continuing review

- Copies of all correspondence with investigators

- Roster of IRB members and their qualifications

- Copies of all SOPs for activities of the IRB

- A copy of correspondence relating a significant new finding that may affect a subject's continuation in the study

The IRB must maintain these records for three years after completion of the research.

Section 3. FDA Actions for Noncompliance by the IRB

FDA has authority to inspect IRBs to assure compliance with their regulatory responsibilities. When the FDA discovers a failure of an IRB to comply, it can undertake a variety of administrative actions to bring the IRB into compliance.

Some of FDA's actions are similar to the compliance actions FDA takes in relation to other regulated parties who are found to be in violation. These actions include: issuing a Form 483 listing observations of deficiencies, sending the IRB a Warning Letter, disqualifying the IRB or its parent institution from participating in the conduct of clinical trials or certain aspects of such studies, disclosing to the public the disqualification, reinstating the IRB or institution when assurances of future compliance are received, and instituting civil or criminal actions depending on the nature of the conduct of the IRB.

Actions available to FDA that are directly related to the clinical trial that may be taken when an IRB is out of compliance include: withholding approval of new studies, prohibiting enrollment of new subjects, terminating ongoing studies, and notifying state and federal regulatory agencies of the noncompliance.

PART 5. INVESTIGATIONAL DEVICE EXEMPTIONS

Section 1. Purpose of the IDE Regulation

Clinical trials are directly controlled and regulated by FDA via the investigational device exemption (IDE) regulation. The primary purpose of the IDE regulation, as stated in the scope section of the IDE regulation, 21 CFR 812.1, is:

> . . . to encourage, to the extent consistent with the protection of the public health and safety and with ethical standards, the discovery and development of useful medical devices intended for human use, and to that end to maintain optimum freedom for scientific investigators in their pursuit of this purpose.

Figure 4.1 is presented in order to put the IDE regulation into perspective along with other major premarketing submissions. It illustrates the

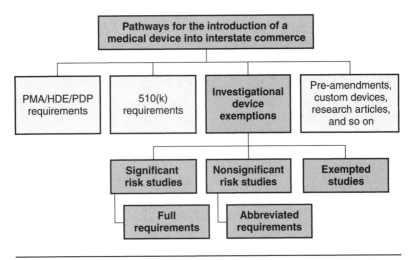

Figure 4.1   Traditional approval/clearance pathways for a medical device.

primary routes that may be taken for the introduction of a medical device into interstate commerce. An approved IDE does not authorize commercial distribution of a medical device; it only authorizes the shipment of the device in interstate commerce for the clinical testing of the device. Chapter 5, Marketing Applications, covers the remaining three boxes in the second tier of Figure 4.1. These other processes allow commercial distribution.

A device that is the subject of an approved IDE may be shipped in interstate commerce, for the purposes approved, without meeting most of the requirements of the law and regulations related to 510(k), PMA, misbranding, registration and listing, performance standards, non-IDE records and reports, GMPs, and others. These various requirements are discussed in other parts of the book.

Section 2. The Role of Engineers and Other Scientists in Clinical Studies

Under state laws, physicians, dentists, and similar healthcare professionals are licensed to treat patients and to "lay hands upon the patient" in rendering their care. This knowledge has led some to believe there is little or no role for engineers and other scientists in the conduct of a clinical trial. However, the conduct of a clinical trial is a complex undertaking that requires the skills and training of many callings, including those of engineers and scientists who have been instrumental in the design and development of the device.

Before a clinical investigator can use a new and complex device, training is required in how the device works, what its limitations are, how to calibrate the device, if that is necessary, what the risks may be, and so on. The designing engineer is frequently the member of the team who provides such instructions.

It may also be important for an engineer to be present during the use of an investigational device to observe the use of the device and the procedures being employed. This involvement of the design team during a clinical trial will provide the opportunity to loop back on design issues and the instructions for use. In fact, one can look at the clinical trial as a natural and necessary extension of the design of the medical device, for it is the clinical trial that represents the ultimate validation of the device design. Participating in the clinical trial will allow further monitoring, review, and feedback on design issues.

Section 3. Applicability

The IDE regulation applies to all clinical investigations of devices to determine safety and effectiveness, unless exempted. This includes studies to support a marketing application for a new device or to collect safety and effectiveness information for a new intended use of a legally marketed device. The IDE regulation also covers a sponsor/investigator who studies an unapproved device or a new intended use of an approved device.

Section 4. Exempted Studies

Studies Exempt from IDE Approval

Every rule seems to have its exceptions, and there are several exceptions to the need for an approved IDE when using the following types of devices or conducting the following types of studies:

- "Pre-amendment" devices in commercial distribution before enactment of the Medical Device Amendments of 1976—excluding transitional devices under an NDA—if used in accordance with the product's labeling, unless the device is being tested for safety and effectiveness (S&E) or substantial equivalence (SE) as the basis for commercial distribution

- Cleared or approved devices, or combinations of legally marketed devices, if used in accordance with the approved label

- Devices shipped for consumer preference testing

- Devices shipped for nonclinical (bench or animal) research
- Veterinary use devices
- Studies performed outside the United States (OUS).
- Custom devices, unless being tested for S&E or SE for commercial distribution
- Devices administered under the emergency use exception
- An in vitro diagnostic device study is exempt if the testing:
  - Is noninvasive
  - Does not require risky invasive sampling
  - Is not intended to introduce energy into the body, and
  - Is not used as a diagnostic procedure without confirmation

Section 5. Significant Risk Studies

The clinical studies to which the IDE regulation is applicable fall into one of two major categories: significant risk (SR) studies or nonsignificant risk (NSR) studies. This distinction is important because an SR study must obtain prior approval from FDA via an IDE before the device can be shipped and a clinical trial initiated, while an NSR study requires IRB approval but does not require FDA's prior approval. NSR study requirements are discussed in section 12 below.

Definition of Significant Risk Study

The clinical trial of a medical device is a significant risk study if the device or its use presents a potentially serious risk to the health, safety, and welfare of a subject and is:

- An implant
- Used in supporting or sustaining human life, or
- Of substantial importance in diagnosing, curing, mitigating, or treating disease or preventing impairment of human health

All other studies are considered to be nonsignificant risk studies.

Requirements for an SR Study

A study that is considered SR requires approval of an IRB and the FDA. The investigational plan and protocol require FDA approval. The investigational plan and protocol are discussed above in part 2, Clinical Trial Design. These approvals are obtained through the submission of an investigational device exemption (IDE) application.

When approved for shipment as an investigational device, the device label must include specified information, including the statement:

> CAUTION—Investigational Device. Limited by Federal (or United States) law to investigational use.

Section 6. Responsibilities of Sponsors

The IDE regulation lists specific responsibilities for sponsors of an SR study. It is important to understand exactly who a "sponsor" is under the regulation. A sponsor means a *person* who initiates a clinical investigation but who does not actually conduct the investigation. A "person," in addition to being a natural human being, may be a corporation, an association, a partnership or sole proprietor, or other "legal" entity. This means that the SR investigation does not have to be sponsored by an individual.

The responsibilities of the sponsor include the following:

- Selecting and contracting with qualified investigators

- Providing to investigators that information necessary to conduct the investigation

- Ensuring proper monitoring

- Ensuring IRB review and approval

- Submitting the IDE to FDA

- Informing the IRB and FDA of any new information

Monitoring Clinical Trials

A sponsor of a clinical trial has an affirmative and independent duty to monitor its clinical trial. Monitoring and auditing are discussed in Chapter 1, part 11, Monitoring and Auditing. There are several methods to accomplish this goal. If a sponsor is a large organization, it may have an internal unit dedicated to this function. Such a group would consist of individuals who have training and experience in the conduct and management of clinical trials. These professionals and scientists frequently have a background in clinical nursing, medicine, biology, and engineering.

A smaller sponsor that does not have the internal capability to monitor its own study can hire a contract research organization (CRO) to monitor the study. Certain CROs specialize in monitoring and auditing clinical trials for a fee.

The purpose of the monitoring is to assure that the study is being conducted in accordance with all of the requirements discussed in this chapter related to clinical trials, including conformance to the approved protocol, all patient protection requirements, IRB rules, and the IDE regulation. This monitoring is conducted primarily through on-site visits by the monitors, who examine the records and documentation of the study to assure that the clinical investigator has discharged the duties discussed below. Monitoring visits and activities have to be documented at each site being monitored.

Data Monitoring Committee

In addition to the general monitoring discussed above, a study sponsor may appoint a data monitoring committee (DMC) to evaluate the outcome data of a clinical trial as they are accumulated. The DMC advises the sponsor regarding the continuing safety of the subjects and on the continuing validity and scientific merit of the trial. In order to bring uniformity to the use of DMCs, FDA published a guidance document entitled *Establishment and Operation of Clinical Trial Data Monitoring Committees* in March 2006. This guidance provides the following description of the use of DMCs:

> DMCs have been a component of some clinical trials since at least the early 1960s. DMCs were initially used primarily in large randomized multicenter trials sponsored by federal agencies, such as the National Institutes of Health (NIH) and the Department of Veterans Affairs (VA) in the U.S. and similar bodies abroad, that targeted improved survival or reduced risk of major morbidity (e.g., acute myocardial infarction) as the primary objective. In 1967, an NIH external advisory group first introduced the concept of a formal committee charged with reviewing the accumulating data as the trial progressed to monitor safety, effectiveness, and trial conduct issues in a set of recommendations to the then–National Heart Institute. (Heart Special Project Committee 'Organization, Review, and Administration of Cooperative Studies [Greenberg Report]: A Report from the Heart Special Project Committee to the National Advisory Heart Council, May 1967'; *Controlled Clinical Trials,* vol. 9, 137–148, 1988.) The recommendation for the establishment of such committees was based on the recognition that interim monitoring of accumulating study data was essential to ensure the ongoing safety of trial participants, but that individuals closely involved with the design and conduct of a trial may not be able to be fully objective in reviewing the interim

data for any emerging concerns. The involvement of expert advisors external to the trial organizers, sponsors, and investigators was intended to ensure that such problems would be addressed in an unbiased way by the trial leadership. The operational and functional aspects of these committees, based on experience over several decades, were discussed in a 1992 NIH workshop (Ellenberg, S., Geller, N., Simon, R., and Yusuf, S. [eds.]: Practical Issues in Data Monitoring of Clinical Trials [workshop proceedings, *Statistics in Medicine,* 12:415–616, 1993]).

Few trials sponsored by the pharmaceutical/medical device industry incorporated DMC oversight until relatively recently. The increasing use of DMCs in industry-sponsored trials is the result of several factors, including:

- The growing number of industry-sponsored trials with mortality or major morbidity endpoints;

- The increasing collaboration between industry and government in sponsoring major clinical trials, resulting in industry trials performed under the policies of government funding agencies, which often require DMCs;

- Heightened awareness within the scientific community of problems in clinical trial conduct and analysis that might lead to inaccurate and/or biased results, especially when early termination for efficacy is a possibility, and need for approaches to protect against such problems;

- Concerns of IRBs regarding ongoing trial monitoring and patient safety in multicenter trials.

The full guidance can be found on the FDA website at:

http://www.fda.gov/RegulatoryInformation/Guidances/ucm127069.htm

The appointment of a DMC will be dependent on the device being studied, its use, the health status of the subjects, and other factors. FDA may request the sponsor to appoint a DMC during the review of the IDE and protocol.

Section 7. Responsibilities of Investigators

A clinical investigator (CI) is defined as an *individual* who actually conducts a clinical investigation. The use of the term "individual" makes it clear that the CI, unlike the sponsor, must be a real person and not an artificial or legal entity. Since the CI is the one in direct contact with the subjects, this requirement assures that there will be individual, as opposed to corporate or organizational, responsibility to the patients as well as the agency. These responsibilities include:

- Ensuring that the investigation is conducted in accordance with the investigator agreement, the protocol, and FDA requirements

- Protecting the rights, safety, and welfare of subjects under his or her care

- Maintaining control of the devices under investigation

- Ensuring that an adequate informed consent is obtained

- Maintaining required records and making required reports to the sponsor, IRB, and FDA

Section 8. FDA Actions on IDE Applications

There are several actions FDA can take in relation to an IDE. FDA may approve the investigation or approve it with modifications. Alternatively, the agency may disapprove the investigation, or it may withdraw the approval of an IDE after initiation of an investigation.

Pre-IDE Meeting

FDA encourages potential IDE applicants to meet with the agency to discuss an upcoming IDE. This pre-IDE meeting provides an opportunity for the sponsor and FDA to discuss the needs of the study and the information FDA will need to approve the IDE. This process can save a great deal of time once an application is received by FDA.

IDE Deficiencies and Amendments

Even with a pre-IDE meeting, deficiencies can, and often do, arise during a thorough IDE review. It may be necessary for the applicant to submit an amendment to the IDE. If the deficiencies are serious enough and correction of the deficiencies will take a significant amount of time, the sponsor may have to submit a new IDE.

IDE Supplements

Once an IDE is approved and the sponsor wants to make a change to the investigation, an IDE supplement may be submitted. There are many reasons why a sponsor might submit such a supplement, which, for example, may include a request for an expansion of the study to additional sites, a request for the enrollment of additional subjects, or a request for the conduct of a live case study for educational purposes. Whatever the reason, FDA will review the request and approve or deny it based on the same types of factors used for the original approval.

IDE Approval

Under the FDCA, a clinical investigation may begin after 30 days of receipt of the IDE by FDA unless FDA takes action before the expiration of the 30 days. Because of this automatic approval provision, FDA always reviews and responds to an IDE within the 30-day review time frame. An IDE has the highest priority for review within CDRH.

Grounds for Denial or Withdrawal of an IDE

The grounds on which FDA may deny approval or withdraw an approval of an IDE are the following:

- Failure of the study to comply with applicable requirements.

- The application or IDE report contained an untrue statement of a material fact.

- Failure on the part of the study to respond to a request for information from FDA.

- The risks are not outweighed by the anticipated benefits.

- Use of the device is unreasonable.

- There were serious inadequacies in the:

  - Report of prior investigations

  - Methods, facilities, and controls for manufacturing, or

  - Monitoring and review of the investigation

Section 9. IDE Prohibitions

Since the approval of an IDE does not constitute approval to commercially market the investigational device, the regulations contain specific prohibitions against conduct that could constitute marketing.

The sponsor may not promote or commercialize the use of the device for medical purposes. Sponsors are permitted to advertise for the purpose of attracting clinical investigators, but such ads may not state or imply that the device is safe or effective for the intended use. These ads are carefully monitored by FDA, and action would be warranted if an ad went beyond acceptable limits.

The representation in any other manner that the device is safe or effective for the purposes for which it is being investigated is strictly prohibited. This would include presentations containing statements of such a nature made by or on behalf of the sponsor or the clinical investigator at a professional meeting at which the progress of the trial or interim results and findings are being reported. It would apply equally to papers published in professional journals.

Another prohibition relates to "unduly prolonging the investigation." Once the necessary number of patients has been treated, FDA expects the sponsor to cease enrollment of new subjects in the trial and, at the completion of the required follow-up periods, to present the results of the investigation in a marketing application. Sometimes, "continued access" to a valuable device may be permitted by FDA during its review of a marketing application, under carefully prescribed conditions. This approach avoids withholding a beneficial product from patients who may benefit from the device while it is under review.

Section 10. Treatment Use of an Investigational Device

There may be times when a device is being studied for a serious disease or condition for which there is no comparable or satisfactory alternative device or other therapy. During the clinical trial or prior to final action on the marketing application, it may be appropriate to use the device in the treatment of patients not in the trial. This would be carried out under the provisions of a treatment IDE.

There are specified criteria that FDA will consider in determining whether to approve a treatment IDE. These criteria are stated as follows in the IDE regulation:

> FDA shall consider the use of an investigational device under a treatment IDE if:
>
> (1) The device is intended to treat or diagnose a serious or immediately life-threatening disease or condition;
>
> (2) There is no comparable or satisfactory alternative device or other therapy available to treat or diagnose that stage of the disease or condition in the intended patient population;
>
> (3) The device is under investigation in a controlled clinical trial for the same use under an approved IDE, or such clinical trials have been completed; and

(4) The sponsor of the investigation is actively pursuing marketing approval/clearance of the investigational device with due diligence.

The regulation goes on to define an "immediately life-threatening" disease as a stage of a disease in which there is a reasonable likelihood that death will occur within a matter of months, or in which premature death is likely, without early treatment.

Even if the basic criteria are met, FDA will not approve the application if other conditions exist. The following selected conditions are among those that would result in denial of the application:

- There is insufficient evidence of safety and effectiveness to support such use.

- The device is intended for an immediately life-threatening disease or condition, and the available scientific evidence, taken as a whole, fails to provide a reasonable basis for concluding that the device:

  - May be effective for its intended use in its intended population, or

  - Would not expose the patients to whom the device is to be administered to an unreasonable and significant additional risk of illness or injury

- The device has received marketing approval/clearance, or a comparable device or therapy becomes available to treat or diagnose the same indication in the same patient population for which the investigational device is being used.

- The clinical investigators named in the treatment IDE are not qualified by reason of their scientific training or experience to use the investigational device for the intended treatment use.

This treatment IDE can be compared to the emergency use exception to the requirements of informed consent discussed above in part 3, Informed Consent. Both of these exceptions are intended to provide the use of an investigational device that may be in the best interest of a patient in need of a special treatment.

Section 11. Confidentiality of IDE Data

FDA will not acknowledge the existence of an IDE before approval of a marketing application for the device unless its existence has been previously disclosed by the sponsor, the clinical investigator, or their agents. If the existence of the IDE is undisclosed, no data or information in the file will be released except for summaries of data upon request as follows:

- When there is a final action on a banned device

- For a report of adverse effects of the device, to a person on whom the device was used

- When the request for information involves an exception to informed consent

Section 12. Nonsignificant Risk (NSR) Studies

The IDE regulation provides for abbreviated requirements for NSR device investigations. In order to qualify for these abbreviated requirements, the following conditions must be met:

- It does not meet the definition of a significant-risk device.

- It is not a banned device.

- It is properly labeled as an investigational device.

- An IRB has approved the investigation as an NSR study.

- Informed consent is obtained.

- The study is properly monitored.

- Specified records are maintained and reports made.

- It complies with prohibitions against promotion.

The primary benefits that accrue under these conditions are that the study does not require FDA approval, and it eliminates most reports to FDA.

Along with the benefits, there are some risks that the sponsor runs. If the sponsor has not previously consulted with FDA, there is a risk that the study may be found by FDA to be an SR study and not an NSR study. In such a case, the sponsor and the IRB may be in violation and subject to a compliance action by the agency.

Another problem that can arise is that the protocol was insufficient for the type of study being conducted. This most likely would be discovered when the sponsor submits a marketing application for FDA review. If FDA finds the protocol to be insufficient, the study may have to be done over. That is why it is always advisable to consult with FDA prior to any investigational device study, even if it is thought to be an NSR study.

PART 6. BIORESEARCH MONITORING

The Bioresearch Monitoring Program (BIMO) is a compliance program designed to monitor all aspects of clinical trials with medical devices. It is a comprehensive, agency-wide program of on-site inspections and data audits designed to monitor all aspects of the conduct and reporting of FDA-regulated research.

As a compliance program, this discussion could have been included in Chapter 7, part 13, QSIT Inspections, because of the similarity between the BIMO and QSIT inspectional processes, or in Chapter 8, Compliance and Enforcement. This discussion also could have been included in Chapter 5, Marketing Applications, because the BIMO reviewers and the findings of BIMO inspections play a critical role in the approval of marketing applications. It is included in this chapter because the BIMO activities are aimed directly at clinical trials and the data they produce. It may be desirable to revisit this section when reading the materials on marketing applications, QSIT inspections, and compliance and enforcement.

The BIMO program impacts and contributes to the review of premarket applications through its oversight of clinical research. It monitors and inspects all aspects of activities related to good clinical practices and marketing applications containing clinical data. Through this program, FDA protects the rights, safety, and welfare of human research subjects, and assures the quality, reliability, and integrity of data collected and submitted to FDA.

Section 1. BIMO Inspections

BIMO Inspection Program

BIMO inspections are conducted pursuant to "compliance programs" that consist of instructions to FDA investigators on the conduct of an inspection for BIMO purposes. The FDA BIMO information web page contains extensive information about the BIMO inspectional programs for IRBs, sponsors, contract research organizations and monitors, and clinical investigators. These programs cover devices, drugs, and biologics. The BIMO information page contains links to these inspection programs and can be found on the FDA website at:

http://www.fda.gov/ora/compliance_ref/bimo/

Under BIMO, field investigators in FDA's District Offices inspect clinical investigators, sponsors, monitors, and CROs, institutional review boards, and nonclinical labs. During these inspections, in addition to the specific items inspected under the compliance program, BIMO investigators will carry out any specific instructions contained in the inspection assignment from CDRH and also observe certain "intangibles" like the corporate culture of the organization, what kind of oversight and control is exercised, patterns of behavior or failures, and the overall attitude of the organization.

Some, but not all, of the specific functions that the BIMO investigator will perform include:

- Checking the investigator's qualifications

- Checking the suitability of the research facility

- Certifying the protocol and the results of the study

- Reviewing the IRB responsible for ensuring the protection of the rights, safety, and well-being of subjects in a study and whether it is adequately constituted to provide assurance of that protection

- Reviewing the IRB's decision to approve or modify and approve the study

- Confirming that the proper device was used in the study

- Checking how informed consent was obtained

- Examining what financial incentives, if any, were provided to subjects or clinical investigators to participate

- Determining how the sponsor monitored the study to ensure that the study was carried out consistently with the protocol

- Looking at a description of how investigators were trained to comply with GCP and to conduct the study in accordance with the protocol

- Checking the presence of a statement that there was adherence to written commitments by investigators to comply with GCP and the protocol

- Checking the accuracy, completeness, and reliability of the data submitted in a premarket submission

BIMO Inspection Form 483

When the inspection is over, the FDA investigator will meet with the organization's management and discuss with them the findings of the inspection.

Significant findings will be presented in writing on a Form 483. Management may respond in writing to the 483 on how they dealt with or will deal with the findings. An adequate response from management to a 483 will contain the following elements:

- An assessment of the root cause of the problem
- An evaluation of the extent of the problem
- The inclusion of any corrective actions to correct the problem
- The plan to institute any preventive actions to avoid recurrence
- Timelines for implementation
- Supporting documentation

BIMO Establishment Inspection Report (EIR)

The BIMO investigator will further prepare an Establishment Inspection Report (EIR), which comprehensively sets forth the details of the inspection and its findings, including exhibits and documents. The EIR will be sent to CDRH for review and final classification. The inspection can result in the one of the following determinations:

1. *No action indicated (NAI).* This determination is based on the fact that there were no objectionable conditions or practices.

2. *Voluntary action indicated (VAI).* This is based on the fact that there were objectionable conditions or practices but not so extensive that they meet the threshold to take or recommend administrative or regulatory action.

3. *Official action indicated (OAI).* In this case, the inspection found serious objectionable conditions, and regulatory action is indicated and recommended.

Based on the final classification of the inspection, FDA will take whatever action is deemed appropriate to rectify the deficiencies, as discussed below in section 3, BIMO Enforcement Actions.

Section 2. Clinical Study Deficiencies

It is instructive to look at the kinds of deficiencies that have been uncovered during BIMO inspections. Table 4.1 identifies the kinds of deficiencies found when inspecting sponsors, clinical investigators, and IRBs during the fiscal year 2008 (October 1, 2007, to September 31, 2008).

Table 4.1   Failures discovered during FY '08 BIMO inspections.

Sponsors failed to:	Investigators failed to:	IRBs failed to provide an adequate:
Control the investigational devices in the study	Follow the investigational plan, the investigator agreement, or the protocol	Initial or continuing review
Secure investigator compliance	Document case histories and device exposure	Frequency of review
Analyze and report adverse events (AEs) and unanticipated AEs	Obtain adequate informed consent	Expedited review
Inform investigators, FDA, or IRB concerning the clinical trial	Control the investigational devices in the study	Records of minutes, membership roster, or study documentation
Monitor the study and follow the protocol or its predetermined plan for data analysis, including selective reporting of studies, study data, or study analyses	Report AEs and unanticipated AEs	Compliance with written procedures for making SR determinations, meeting quorum, reports on noncompliance, and frequency of review
Obtain a signed investigator agreement	Obtain FDA/IRB approval to conduct study	SR determination
Obtain an acceptable informed consent		Membership roster

Section 3. BIMO Enforcement Actions

Based on the findings of the BIMO inspection, there are a variety of review decisions and administrative and legal actions available to FDA. The list is long, and the major actions are listed below. Most of these actions are generally applicable to other violations of the FDCA and regulations, as well as clinical trials, and are discussed in Chapter 8, Compliance and Enforcement. Some are only applicable to marketing applications, and they are discussed in Chapter 5, Marketing Applications.

- Untitled Letter

- Warning Letter

- Deficiency letter

- IRB restrictions on new studies or subjects

- Rejection of data

- Application Integrity Policy action

- Application withdrawal

- Disqualification of the clinical investigator

- Civil money penalties

- Detention/seizure

- Injunction

- Criminal prosecution

- Consent agreement/decree

PART 7. IMPORTING AND EXPORTING MEDICAL DEVICES FOR INVESTIGATIONAL USE

This part deals with importing and exporting an investigational medical device. Importing or exporting a medical device for marketing is covered in Chapter 5, part 4, Importing and Exporting Medical Devices for Commercial Distribution. In addition to the requirements set forth in section 1 and section 2 below, certain record-keeping requirements also apply to device exporters.

Section 1. Importing an Investigational Device

From time to time a question arises concerning the importation of an investigational device. A person may want to import an investigational device for the purpose of obtaining U.S. data on the device for submission to FDA in a marketing application. Data from a study conducted outside the United States are acceptable in a marketing application, provided they meet the requirements set forth earlier in this chapter in part 1, section 2, International Guidelines for Medical Research. Data from a United States study generally are not mandatory in an application for marketing approval but they can facilitate the process. Sometimes a U.S. study arm can confirm the findings of a foreign-based clinical study.

In order to import an investigational device, the person importing the device must meet all IDE requirements, serve as the U.S. agent of the foreign exporter, serve as the sponsor of the investigation, or provide assurances that someone else serves as agent and sponsor. Failure to meet these requirements would render the device adulterated or misbranded and subject to embargo by FDA.

Section 2. Exporting an Investigational Device

There are times when a person may want to export an investigational device to another country for the purpose of carrying on a clinical study. This may be desirable if, for example, the incidence of the disease for which the device is intended occurs at a higher rate in a particular region of the world and there is a likelihood of enrolling more subjects for the study.

In other cases, the foreign government may find the device acceptable for medical use in its country based on its own evaluation of available data even though the device has not yet been approved for marketing by FDA. The FDA is careful in issuing export permits because it is the policy of the United States not to "dump" unsafe or ineffective products on other countries that may not have the benefit of an agency like FDA to protect its citizens from unproven devices.

An investigational device (as well as a device that lacks a necessary PMA or does not comply with an applicable performance standard, or a banned device) can be exported with FDA approval, that is, an export permit, or it can be exported without FDA approval if, among other conditions, it (1) has marketing authorization in the importing country, (2) complies with the laws of the country to which it is being exported, (3) accords to the specifications of the foreign purchaser, (4) is in a shipping package labeled for export, (5) is not sold or offered for sale in domestic commerce, and (6) complies with certain manufacturing, labeling, and promotional requirements. The exporter of a device without an FDA export permit is required to notify FDA when the exporter first begins to export the device.

PART 8. NATIONAL CLINICAL TRIALS DATA BANK

This discussion of the national Clinical Trials Data Bank is included in this chapter on investigational devices rather than including it in Chapter 5, Marketing Applications, because the primary purpose of this requirement is to make information about clinical trials available to the general public. Its enforcement happens to occur when a marketing application is submitted to FDA, and that aspect is discussed below in section 3, FDA Certification.

Section 1. Background and Purpose

There has been a movement in the United States for some years for the government to make information about ongoing clinical trials publicly available so that individuals may have the opportunity to join a clinical trial as a subject and obtain needed treatment or to find out new information about the disease or condition being treated.

To meet this need, a Clinical Trials Data Bank was established by section 113 of the Food and Drug Administration Modernization Act (FDAMA) of 1997. Section 113 of FDAMA creates a public resource for information on studies of drugs for serious or life-threatening diseases and conditions conducted under FDA's investigational new drug (IND) regulations. The Food and Drug Administration Amendments Act (FDAAA) of 2007 amended and expanded the use of the data bank to include medical device trials.

The law requires the registration of clinical trials with the data bank that is maintained at the National Institutes of Health. ClinicalTrials.gov is a registry of federally and privately supported clinical trials conducted in the United States and around the world. ClinicalTrials.gov provides information about a trial's purpose, who may participate, locations, and phone numbers for more details.

Clinical trials must be registered in accordance with 402(j) of the PHSA. Clinical trials are registered with ClinicalTrials.gov via a web-based data entry system called the Protocol Registration System (PRS). More information on this process can be accessed at:

> http://www.clinicaltrials.gov

Also, the NIH Fact Sheet entitled "Registration at ClinicalTrials.gov: As Required by Public Law 110-85, Title VIII" explains the registration system for clinical trials in the ClinicalTrials.gov database at:

> http://prsinfo.clinicaltrials.gov/s801-fact-sheet.pdf

Section 2. Exempted Clinical Trials

This registration requirement does not apply to all types of clinical trials. According to the act, Section 402(j)(1)(A)(ii), an "applicable device clinical trial" is:

> . . . a prospective clinical study of health outcomes comparing an intervention with a device subject to Section 510(k), 515, or 520(m) of the Federal Food, Drug, and Cosmetic Act against a control in human subjects . . . and a pediatric post-market surveillance as required under Section 522 of the Federal Food, Drug, and Cosmetic Act.

It does not encompass:

> . . . a small clinical trial to determine the feasibility of a device, or a clinical trial to test prototype devices where the primary outcome measure relates to feasibility and not to health outcomes . . . .

Section 3. FDA Certification

In order to assure that clinical trials have been registered, a certification must accompany the following marketing submissions for medical devices to FDA:

- Original 510(k)s
- Original PMAs
- Panel-track PMA supplements
- 180-day PMA supplements with clinical data
- Original HDEs
- Pediatric post-market surveillance of devices required by FDA in an approval order

The applicant must make one of the following certifications before FDA will review and approve the foregoing submissions:

A. I certify that the requirements of 42 U.S.C. § 282(j), Section 402(j) of the Public Health Service Act, enacted by 121 Stat. 823, Public Law 110-85, do not apply because the application/submission which this certification accompanies does not reference any clinical trial.

B. I certify that the requirements of 42 U.S.C. § 282(j), Section 402(j) of the Public Health Service Act, enacted by 121 Stat. 823, Public Law 110-85, do not apply to any clinical trial referenced in the application/submission which this certification accompanies.

C. I certify that the requirements of 42 U.S.C. § 282(j), Section 402(j) of the Public Health Service Act, enacted by 121 Stat.

823, Public Law 110-85, apply to one or more of the clinical trials referenced in the application/submission which this certification accompanies and that those requirements have been met.

PART 9. EXERCISES

1. What is the meaning of "good clinical practices"?

2. Name the major regulations governing clinical trials.

3. Search the CODEX Web site and briefly identify the most important and most used international standards applicable to clinical trials.

4. Why is financial disclosure important in the conduct of human studies?

5. What is the purpose of a clinical study?

6. When is informed consent required?

7. What is the purpose of an IRB in a clinical trial?

8. When are the requirements of the IDE regulation applicable to a clinical trial?

9. What is the difference between a significant risk study and a nonsignificant risk study?

10. What is the Bioresearch Monitoring Program and what is its purpose?

5

Marketing Applications

THE SCOPE OF THIS CHAPTER

There are four types of marketing submissions that are required for the commercial distribution of a medical device in the United States: a Premarket Notification, or 510(k), a Premarket Approval (PMA) application, a product development protocol (PDP), and a humanitarian device exemption (HDE). The approval of a PMA, its associated applications such as the PDP and HDE, or the clearance of a 510(k), authorize the commercial distribution of the device for the diagnosis or treatment of a disease, illness, or condition in humans.

Clinical data are required for PMAs, HDEs, and PDPs, and for some 510(k)s. For the purpose of gathering the requisite data, clinical trial design considerations and good clinical practices, informed consent, and IRBs are discussed in Chapter 4, Clinical Trials, along with IDE applications.

The Office of Device Evaluation (ODE) and the Office of In Vitro Diagnostic Evaluation and Safety (OIVD) in FDA's Center for Devices and Radiological Health (CDRH) have the primary responsibility for managing the processing and approval or clearance of premarket submissions for medical devices. These offices process a great number of premarket submissions each year. To illustrate the volume of submissions received and processed, Table 5.1 lists the number of major submissions received and completed by these offices for the fiscal years indicated in the table. The table does not, however, include all submissions managed during those time periods, such as amendments and 513(g) inquiries.

EARLY PLANNING

Once the design of the device, it's nonclinical testing, and the clinical trials are complete, it is time to submit a marketing application to FDA. The

Table 5.1 Major submissions received and completed by fiscal year.

Office of Device Evaluation (for FY 2008)
Office of In Vitro Diagnostic Devices (for FY 2005)

Type of submission	Number received by ODE	Number completed by ODE	Number received by OIVD	Number completed by OIVD
Original PMAs	26	16	6	11
PMA supplements	1448	630	84	28
Original IDEs	216	215	6	6
IDE supplements	4409	4369	23	0
510(k)s	3363	3238	520	23
Original HDEs	3	2	1	0
HDE supplements	40	42	0	0
Totals	9505	8512	640	572

end goal of all of these efforts is to obtain the information and data that will be required to obtain marketing approval or clearance for a new medical device. Hence, the requirements of the device evaluation programs are the controlling factors in performing the designing and testing of a device intended for medical use. It is important to know as early as possible in the design and development process what FDA will expect in a marketing application so that all the right steps can be taken.

As an example, some of the types of early questions that may be useful to have an answer to could include:

- What special design features will be expected for the device under development?

- What type of nonclinical testing will the agency expect?

- In the case of clinical testing, what type of study will be required, how many patients will be needed, what end points will work, and so on?

- What statistical data and analysis will FDA be looking for?

Failure to prepare the marketing application properly can result in a waste of time and money. Therefore, it is critical to discuss, at the earliest time possible, the development plans with the appropriate review division in CDRH to obtain as much guidance as possible. The agency encourages meetings during the development process and looks forward to pre-IDE meetings, pre-PMA meetings, and other interim meetings as may be necessary. Early and adequate communication can save valuable resources for both the agency and the device developer.

The FDA application, review, and approval process may at times seem daunting, but it is not an unfamiliar process. In fact, the FDA review process can be compared to the process used by peer review journals in accepting a scientific article for publication. Table 5.2 compares these two processes.

Table 5.2   Comparison of professional journal publications versus submission of applications to FDA for approval.

Publish research results in a professional journal	Submit an application to FDA for marketing approval/clearance
Conduct the research, gather the data, analyze it, draw conclusions, and write and submit the article to a peer review journal for publication.	Conduct the research, gather the data, analyze it, draw conclusions, and write and submit the application to FDA for approval/clearance.
Article is distributed for peer review.	Submission is reviewed by an FDA review team.
Journal sends to author comments, challenges, objections submitted by expert reviewers.	FDA sends to applicant a request for additional information or a deficiency letter prepared by the review team.
Author sends revised draft to journal based on the reviewers' comments.	Applicant sends amendments to the submission to FDA responding to reviewers' comments.
Journal submits new draft to experts for review.	FDA reviews the application with amendments. The submission may be reviewed by an FDA advisory panel.
If the redraft is adequate, the article is published.	If there is sufficient evidence that the device is substantially equivalent or reasonably safe and effective, the device is cleared or approved for marketing.

The FDA review process, however, will differ in its detail and intensity, which is not insignificant.

PART 1. GLOBAL MARKETING APPLICATION CONCEPTS

The global concepts discussed in this part deal with substantive issues and process issues that have general applicability in the review and evaluation of all types of marketing submissions discussed in this chapter. Each of the following issues is discussed in this part to avoid duplication of the material for each of the marketing submissions covered in subsequent parts of this chapter:

- Overview of the premarket review process—section 1

- Valid scientific evidence—section 2

- Labeling and unapproved uses—section 3

- Advisory committee review and outside expertise—section 4

- Intermediate FDA actions during the review process—section 5

- Financial disclosure—section 6

- Data integrity—section 7

- Bioresearch monitoring—section 8

- CDRH electronic copy initiative—section 9

- Medical device user fees—section 10

CDRH has issued two preliminary reports that may affect the discussions contained in this chapter in particular and other chapters to a lesser extent. Some of the scientific topics listed above, such as "valid scientific evidence" and "labeling and unapproved uses" may be affected in the future. Since these reports arose within the context of the 510(k) program, they are discussed below in part 2, section 9, Upcoming 510(k) Program Changes.

Section 1. Overview of the Premarket Review Process

The premarket review and evaluation process is a peer review–type system applied to all types of marketing submissions, including 510(k)s, PMAs, PDPs, HDEs, and the various amendments and supplemental submissions. The review process takes into account scientific, medical, and regulatory considerations related to the device and the application in determining whether to approve or clear the submission. The review depends, for example, on the particular device, its intended uses, its potential risks, the type of data presented, and any special manufacturing methods. Therefore, any particular submission review may involve internal and external scientific, medical, and technical experts and internal regulatory experts from the pre-market, post-market, and compliance components of the CDRH.

Application Review within CDRH

There are two offices within the Center for Devices and Radiological Health that have the main responsibility for the review of marketing applications: the Office of Device Evaluation and the Office of In Vitro Diagnostic Evaluation and Safety.

ODE comprises five review divisions with approximately 350 reviewers. OIVD is divided into three divisions of approximately 60 reviewers. The review divisions are structured with branches organized by therapeutic or diagnostic specialty areas.

Device Review Teams

Review teams are assigned the task of evaluating marketing submissions. The teams are usually composed of the following individuals:

- Lead reviewer

- Medical/clinical reviewer

- Engineer (biomedical, material, mechanical, electrical, and so on)

- Statistician

- Patient labeling reviewer

- Manufacturing reviewer

- Bioresearch Monitoring (BIMO) reviewer

- Other specialists, as appropriate, in areas such as toxicology, microbiology, biocompatibility, software, human factors, optics, veterinary medicine, and so on

During or after the analysis and evaluation of the marketing submission, the review team or consulting specialists will prepare a "review memo," which will be presented to division and center management. There may be more than one review memo, or specialized memos dealing with particular issues like electrical safety, statistical analysis, composition of the study population, integrity of the data, biocompatibility, or any topic that may have special applicability to the review of the submission. Review memos may be prepared by individuals with special expertise on a particular issue. CDRH has listed some review memos on the web page entitled "Premarket Approval (PMA) Summary Review Memos for 180-Day Design Changes," and they can be accessed by selecting any of the links appearing in the list.

> http://www.fda.gov/AboutFDA/CentersOffices/CDRH/
> CDRHTransparency/ucm206289.htm

Previously, review memos had not been made publicly available. This web page is the initial posting of review memos and, hopefully, it will be expanded by the agency to include all review memos over time. This is an important development because it will give the public insight into the way the agency makes its approval decisions.

Risk-Based System

The law gives FDA the flexibility to calibrate its regulatory rigor to the level of the potential risk posed by the product. For example, a device that poses a low risk to a patient, usually a Class I or Class II device, may be cleared for marketing via a 510(k) while a device that poses a greater risk to patients, usually a Class III device, would have to pass the more rigorous review of a PMA. There are exceptions to this general rule that would be made on a case-by-case basis.

Section 2. Valid Scientific Evidence

United States Data

In the review of marketing submissions, the evidence required to establish safety and effectiveness or substantial equivalence may vary according to the characteristics of a device, its conditions of use, the existence and adequacy of warnings and other restrictions, and the extent of experience with its use. The evidence must be of a nature such that qualified experts can fairly and responsibly conclude that there is reasonable assurance of the safety and effectiveness of the device under its conditions of use or that the device is substantially equivalent to a predicate device. All of this evidence must constitute "valid scientific evidence," which may include:

- Well-controlled investigations

- Partially controlled studies

- Studies and objective trials without matched controls

- Well-documented case histories conducted by qualified experts

- Reports of significant human experience with a marketed device

- Statistical analysis

The following types of information are not considered to be valid scientific evidence:

- Isolated case reports

- Random experience

- Reports lacking sufficient details to permit scientific evaluation

- Unsubstantiated opinions

Foreign Data

Data gathered outside the United States (OUS) may be used in support of an FDA marketing submission. It may consist of nonclinical or clinical data and information. An applicant may use OUS data in any of the marketing applications discussed in this chapter, including a 510(k), PMA, PDP, and HDE.

OUS data must meet the same standard as U.S. data and constitute valid scientific evidence in the same manner as data gathered in the United States. However, the OUS data must have been gathered in a study that was conducted in accordance with the Declaration of Helsinki or the laws and regulations of the country in which the study was conducted. If the study was conducted in accordance with the laws of the country, the PMA applicant is required to explain to FDA in detail the differences between the laws of the country and the Declaration of Helsinki.

Section 3. Labeling and Unapproved Uses

Labeling

Medical devices must contain appropriate labeling. Labeling includes the label on the package as well as supplementary information in package inserts, instruction manuals, and other information provided with the device. For medical devices, labeling, in general, must include:

- The name and place of manufacturer, packer, distributor

- The intended use

- Adequate directions for use, and

- It must not contain any misleading statements

Labeling should include information about risks, precautions, warnings, potential adverse reactions, and so on.

Human Factors Evaluation of Labeling

FDA offers an extensive guidance on labeling of medical devices entitled "Human Factors Principles for Medical Device Labeling," which can be found at:

> http://www.fda.gov/downloads/MedicalDevices/Device
> RegulationandGuidance/GuidanceDocuments/UCM095300.pdf

This guidance covers the organization, format, and content of labeling, especially from the point of view of the user's proper understanding and safe and effective use of the device. Of particular interest from the device design standpoint is the information concerning the testing of the labeling to make sure it is appropriate to the intended audience. In this regard it states:

> Labeling for a medical device that has been approved by FDA should undergo premarket testing and evaluation. Pretesting involves the systematic collection of data from members of the intended user group on various characteristics of the labeling. Pretesting can identify specific strengths and weaknesses of labeling. Use the findings from pretesting to improve labeling before the device is brought to market.
>
> Pretests of labeling should focus on one or more of the following areas: user comprehension, user performance, acceptability, and credibility. Focus on the characteristics of the intended user group to make the labeling most effective for them. A major shortcoming of much medical device labeling is that it has not been written with the target users in mind. Consequently, users have often misunderstood or been unable to comprehend labeling. Several methods can be used to pretest medical device labeling, including focus group interviews, in-depth individual interviews, questionnaires, and readability testing. Most often, some combination of these methods must be used to develop the most effective labeling possible.

Adequate Directions for Use

All regulated products must bear adequate directions for use to allow the safe use of the product. The requirement that a device be labeled with adequate directions for use is intended for devices that are marketed directly to the public for personal use. These products are referred to as "over-the-counter," or OTC, products. If a device can not be labeled with adequate directions for use, then the sale of the device must be restricted to professional supervision. In such a case, the product would become a "prescription device" or a "restricted device." Such devices are used under the supervision of, or on the order of, a health care practitioner licensed to administer or dispense such products. This so called "exemption" from adequate directions for use also applies to in vitro diagnostic products and devices for processing, repackaging, and manufacturing.

Restricted or prescription devices must contain professional instructions for use. These instructions may consist of a relatively simple package insert, or they may be very extensive for complex devices and consist of an instruction manual. Sometimes, certain devices require special labeling that can often be found in the classification regulation for the specific device. FDA may, at the time of approval, require special labeling, warnings, cautions, and other information necessary for the safe and effective use of the device. The labeling for a device approved under a PMA must be approved by FDA, as well as labeling for devices cleared under a 510(k).

Labeling Review

The exact wording in the labeling of a medical device can be tricky, especially if the instructions are intended for the home use of an OTC device. There can be a wide range of linguistic sophistication among lay users that has to be taken into account when reviewing proposed language for a label. Language issues may arise in prescription labeling as well as OTC labeling. CDRH employs individuals who specialize in dealing with communication issues that may arise in the labeling of all types of medical devices, both restricted and OTC devices, and they play a vital role in reviewing proposed labeling for devices under review by CDRH.

Unapproved Uses

A PMA will contain the full labeling for the device, and a 510(k), depending on the device, will include the full labeling or the indications for use. This then becomes the official labeling for the product. The manufacturer may not promote or advertise the device, including oral representations by sales representatives, for a use that differs from the approved labeling, including different indications for use, a different dosage, use in a different patient population, or use of a different mode of administration.

Different uses such as these that deviate from the official labeling would be "unapproved uses," which may result in the misbranding or adulteration of the device and be subject to an agency enforcement action.

Using a device for an unapproved use by a physician will generally have no effect on the physician or the device. Physicians who use the device are exempted by law from the labeling requirements if it is done in the course of their professional practice. However, if they attempt to redistribute the device or sell it to other practitioners for an unapproved use, the exemption would not apply and they would have to fulfill the same responsibilities as a manufacturer or distributor.

Section 4. Advisory Committee Review and Outside Expertise

External Expertise

The CDRH uses various outside experts to supplement and broaden its internal expertise in carrying out its responsibilities. One source of obtaining outside expertise is through collaboration with the clinical community and professional groups. This source is limited to general policy and procedure issues that may be discussed in public forums, because only government employees or "special" government employees (SGEs) may be given access to confidential and trade secret information contained in marketing applications. To accommodate this requirement, CDRH has turned to SGEs through several programs to obtain the support needed.

Medical Device Fellowship Program

The Medical Device Fellowship Program (MDFP) is a program that appoints "fellows" of varying scientific and clinical specialties to join the CDRH staff for specified periods of time. Since the inception of the fellowship program, about 170 participants have joined the Center's staff through various technology transfer requests and agreements such as memorandums of understanding (MOU), Cooperative Research and Development Agreements (CRADAs), grants, Interagency Agreements (IAA), and Joint Fellowship Agreements (JFA). These fellows apply their expertise to the review and analysis of scientific and medical issues presented during the review of applications and to the development of guidance for the industry and FDA staff.

Medical Devices Advisory Panels

The major source of outside input from technical experts is through the FDA advisory committee system. The Medical Devices Advisory Committee is divided into 18 panels, each of which deals with a specialty area of medical devices as listed below.

- Anesthesiology and respiratory therapy devices
- Circulatory system devices
- Clinical chemistry and clinical toxicology devices
- Dental products

- Dispute resolution

- Ear, nose, and throat devices

- Gastroenterology and urology devices

- General and plastic surgery devices

- General hospital and personal use devices

- Hematology and pathology devices

- Immunology devices

- Microbiology devices

- Molecular and clinical genetics devices

- Neurological devices

- Obstetrics and gynecology devices

- Ophthalmic devices

- Orthopedic and rehabilitation devices

- Radiological devices

Panel Members

The Medical Devices Advisory Committee is composed of SGEs appointed as voting members or consultants. The advisory committee has a maximum of 159 standing members within the 18 panels. Voting members are selected by the agency based on their expertise in clinical and administrative medicine, engineering, the biological and physical sciences, and statistics and other necessary professions. A consumer representative is nominated by a consumer nominating group, and an industry representative is nominated by industry. There may also be a temporary voting member added to a particular panel as needed to provide the expertise required due to the absence of a standing member or to comprise a quorum. An FDA staff member serves as the executive secretary to each panel.

Panel Meetings

During panel meetings and panel deliberations, the panel will consider the merits of an application under review. Information and issues concerning the application and other supporting materials assembled in a "panel pack" will have been previously mailed to the panel members well in advance of the meeting. This panel pack is also made available to the public. For an example of a panel pack, see the following FDA web page entitled "2011

Meeting Materials of the Circulatory System Devices Panel," which contains links to the documents sent to the panel in preparation for an upcoming meeting.

> http://www.fda.gov/AdvisoryCommittees/CommitteesMeeting
> Materials/MedicalDevices/MedicalDevicesAdvisoryCommittee/
> CirculatorySystemDevicesPanel/ucm240575.htm

Both the applicant whose application is under discussion and the FDA have the opportunity to make a presentation to and respond to questions from the panel. The panel then discusses or debates the issues related to the application.

All panel meetings are open to the public unless trade secret or confidential commercial information is discussed. The portion of the meeting at which nondisclosable information is discussed will be closed to the public. About 30 minutes from the end of every open panel meeting, members of the public may make presentations to the panel.

During the panel's deliberations, FDA will make a final summation, and the applicant will have an opportunity to do the same. When the panel has finished its discussions, the panel will vote on its recommendation to FDA and the meeting will be adjourned.

Panel Recommendations

The panel may make any of the following recommendations to FDA:

- *Approval, without conditions.* This occurs when the panel has no prohibitive concerns about approving the device as presented.

- *Approvable, with conditions.* In this case, the panel thinks the device is approvable but needs, for example, further analysis of existing data, post-approval studies, user or patient training, or labeling revisions. All conditions are voted on prior to the vote on the main approval motion.

- *Not approvable.* This can occur when the panel sees major problems with the nonclinical testing or clinical trial. The panel may think there is a need for a new clinical study. This may be due, for example, to insufficient safety and effectiveness data or inadequate patient follow-up.

Posted Panel Meeting Information

In addition to the panel pack, FDA makes available other panel materials to the public. A brief summary of the meeting is posted on the FDA website within a business day of the meeting. It describes the panel vote and any recommendations.

Panel summary minutes are available within 60 to 90 days of the meeting. This document summarizes matters discussed, the FDA questions addressed, and the panel's conclusions and recommendations.

A complete transcript or recording of the entire meeting is made by a court reporter. The transcript of the open, public portion of the meeting is available 30 to 60 days after the meeting from the transcription company, but the transcript of a closed session is not made publicly available.

FDA Actions on Panel Recommendations

Panel recommendations are not binding on the agency. FDA will consider the panel recommendations in deciding whether to approve or disapprove the application under consideration.

Section 5. Intermediate FDA Actions During the Review Process

During the review of marketing applications, there are several actions that may be taken by FDA. For example, the agency may need a clarification of studies, data, or analyses, or the labeling or intended use may raise questions. If the issue is of a minor nature, a reviewer may telephone the applicant for clarification. At other times they may issue a "minor deficiency" letter or a letter requesting additional information. These issues are usually easily resolved.

When more-significant issues arise, the agency will issue a "major deficiency" letter. These letters present issues that can not be answered easily and usually take a significant amount of time to resolve. For example, the application may need new or additional nonclinical or clinical studies. The application may contain insufficient safety or effectiveness data or insufficient patient follow-up.

Depending on the severity of the deficiency, an amendment to the application may be required or, in some cases, a new application may have to be submitted. No final action on an application can be taken until all questions concerning the application are resolved.

Section 6. Financial Disclosure

All clinical data submitted in marketing applications must be complete, accurate, truthful, and unbiased. The agency can then rely on the data in making its evaluations for marketing. If the data in a marketing application are not reliable, FDA's evaluation of the data would not be valid and its decision making would be impaired. To produce reliable application data, clinical trials must be objective and free of bias. The objectivity of the investigators should not be clouded by conflicts of interest that might affect the reliability of the data.

To provide protection against hidden financial arrangements that might raise questions about the objectivity and impartiality of the data in the application, FDA regulations require applicants submitting clinical trial data to (1) include a certification (Form 3454) listing all clinical investigators and their financial interests, and (2) submit a disclosure statement (Form FDA 3455) for each clinical investigator included in the certification disclosing the financial interests of the investigator, attesting to the absence of financial interests of the investigator, or stating that the applicant used due diligence in trying to get the required information.

Financial interests of an investigator can call into question the objectivity of the trial. See discussion of bias in clinical research in Chapter 4, part 1, section 5, Bias and Financial Conflicts of Interest.

Section 7. Data Integrity

General Rule

It is a crime to make a false or misleading statement of a material fact to any federal agency. The relevant part of the U.S. criminal code states, at 18 USC 1001:

> (a) Except as otherwise provided in this section, whoever, in any matter within the jurisdiction of the executive, legislative, or judicial branch of the Government of the United States, knowingly and willfully—
>
> (1) falsifies, conceals, or covers up by any trick, scheme, or device a material fact;
>
> (2) makes any materially false, fictitious, or fraudulent statement or representation; or
>
> (3) makes or uses any false writing or document knowing the same to contain any materially false, fictitious, or fraudulent statement or entry;
>
> shall be fined under this title, imprisoned not more than 5 years or . . . .

This law has general applicability to statements made to any branch of the federal government, including written, verbal, or electronic statements. Accordingly, it is applicable to submissions to and communications with FDA.

FDA's Application Integrity Policy

The validity of data is especially important in the medical device review process. FDA decisions depend on reliable data, and information that is complete, accurate, and truthful. This not only assures better decision making but also assures that the review process is fair, impartial, secure, and reliable.

To enhance the integrity of its various review processes (medical devices, drugs, biologics, foods, and veterinarian products), FDA adopted the Application Integrity Policy (AIP). This policy is based on the agency's general review authorities rather than Title 18, as quoted above. Thus, it represents an administrative remedy as opposed to criminal prosecution. However, if an applicant submits a false or misleading statement of a material fact, the FDA Office of Criminal Investigations may, concurrently with the AIP action, institute its own criminal investigation. The Application Integrity Policy can be found at the following FDA web page:

http://www.fda.gov/downloads/ICECI/EnforcementActions/
ApplicationIntegrityPolicy/UCM072631.pdf

Under this policy, a "wrongful act" and an "untrue statement of material fact" are defined in the AIP, section 1-1-3, in the following manner:

> A wrongful act is any act that may subvert the integrity of the review process. A wrongful act includes, but is not limited to, submitting a fraudulent application, offering or promising a bribe or illegal gratuity, or making an untrue statement of material fact. A wrongful act also includes submitting data that are otherwise unreliable due to, for example, a pattern of errors whether caused by incompetence, negligence, or a practice such as inadequate standard operating procedures or a system-wide failure to ensure the integrity of data submissions . . . .
>
> An "untrue statement of material fact" is a false statement, misstatement, or omission of a fact. A determination that an untrue statement is material is necessary for purposes of invoking the AIP. The Center should make a written determination. This determination may involve discussions with OCC.

Wrongful acts are actionable by FDA. The agency may discover a wrongful act through various means. Information may come from: tips from an anonymous or known informant, current or former company employees, former business partners of the applicant, patients, other federal agencies (Securities and Exchange Commission, Federal Trade Commission, Centers for Medicare and Medicaid Services), suspicious data found during scientific or clinical review, or observations made during preapproval inspections. A wrongful act may be evidenced in a document, including informal documents such as correspondence or memoranda, or verbally, such as in telephone conversations or in meetings.

This information also may be discovered during a BIMO inspection of the manufacturer or sponsor, at a clinical site, or during the inspection of a CRO. When unreliable data are suspected, the agency will conduct data and system audits and examine company internal documents.

Some of the kinds of problems that have resulted in data integrity actions include:

- Falsification of specific data or an entire submission

- Omission of relevant and important data and information

- Inability to account for patient populations

- Inability to account for investigational devices

- Failure to maintain adequate investigational records

- Failure to follow the protocol

- Unreported changes to the investigational device

Remedies for Invalid Data under AIP

The remedies available when false or misleading data are discovered in an application are serious. Correction of the problem can be very expensive for the company in terms of time, money, and staff resources. Public notice of an agency action based on the Application Integrity Policy can also be damaging to the company's reputation. The options available to FDA include:

- Denial or withdrawal of approval of an application

- Disqualification of the data for:

  - Individual subjects

  - An entire study site, or

  - The entire data set in the study

- Issuance of an AIP or Integrity Hold (IH) letter

- Civil or criminal prosecution

Disqualifications and civil or criminal prosecutions are discussed in Chapter 8, part 2, Compliance Actions and Penalties. AIP and IH letters are discussed immediately below.

AIP and IH Letters

Issuance of an IH or AIP letter is an administrative action. In essence, these letters inform a company that the agency will no longer conduct a scientific review of one or more of its submissions until the company undertakes certain corrective actions, including:

- An independent, third-party audit of the data in the application

- An independent, third-party audit of the company's system, policies, and procedures for conducting testing, maintaining records, preparing applications, and other activities for submissions to FDA

- The preparation of an acceptable corrective and preventive action (CAPA) plan that will provide assurance that the data in submissions to FDA will be complete, accurate, and truthful

Auditing is covered in Chapter 1, part 11, Monitoring and Auditing. A discussion of the requirements for an acceptable CAPA plan can be found in Chapter 7, part 8, Corrective and Preventive Actions.

The major difference between an IH and an AIP letter is that the former applies to one application and the latter results from data integrity problems in more than one application. Table 5.3 compares these two letters.

Table 5.3   AIP versus IH letters.

AIP letter	IH letter
Defers scientific review on *all* submissions	Defers scientific review on *one* submission
Requires data audit	Requires data audit
Requires system audit	Requires system audit
Requires CAPA	Requires CAPA
Stops the review clock until the AIP is removed (usually 1–2 years)	Stops the review clock until the IH is removed (usually 1–2 years)
Uses separate AIP boilerplate	Uses deficiency letter boilerplate
Signed by center director	Signed by division director

Section 8. Bioresearch Monitoring

The Bioresearch Monitoring Program (BIMO) impacts and contributes to the review of premarket applications through its oversight of clinical research. It monitors and inspects all aspects of activities related to good clinical practices and marketing applications containing clinical data. Since the main purpose of the BIMO program is to monitor clinical research, a comprehensive discussion of the BIMO program is included in Chapter 4, part 6, Bioresearch Monitoring.

BIMO reviewers and the findings of BIMO inspections, however, play a critical role in the approval of marketing applications. A BIMO compliance officer is a member of the application review team. The BIMO reviewers advise the review team on the (1) oversight of the study and its monitoring plans, (2) adequacy of subject protection and other GCP issues, and (3) clinical sites to be inspected. They translate any identified GCP concerns into the inspection assignment and report back to the review team on the inspection results during and after the inspection.

Section 9. CDRH Electronic Copy Initiative

There has been an effort on the part of the FDA to automate as much of its operations as possible, including the premarket review program. One aspect of this effort that has received attention is the use of electronic submissions. The program is being expanded on a continuous basis. At the present time an e-copy may be submitted for any premarket submission: 510(k), PMA, IDE, HDE. The e-copy must be an exact duplicate of the hard-copy premarket submission in electronic form (CD/DVD). FDA specifies the format that is needed for PDF files, SAS, XPORT, XML, and other specific file types.

When received by FDA, the document is immediately loaded into their electronic system. The electronic copy then replaces one of the required paper copies. There are several benefits when applicants submit an e-copy. The file is available immediately for use by the review staff, and the navigational tools facilitate the review process. This can help shorten the time it takes to review the application and results in a faster final decision. Everyone benefits from a shorter review time: the manufacturer gets to market sooner, the patients have a new technology available for their care, and the agency saves processing time and money.

More information on electronic submissions is available at:

http://www.fda.gov/MedicalDevices/DeviceRegulationand
Guidance/HowtoMarketYourDevice/PremarketSubmissions/
ucm134508.htm

Section 10. Medical Device User Fees

Congress has authorized FDA to charge submitters a fee for the processing of premarket applications for medical devices through FY 2012. Table 5.4 itemizes the major fees in effect for FY 2010. These fees change from time to time. Column "SB < $1M" contains the fees for small businesses making less than $1,000,000.

These user fees allow FDA to make significant improvements in the medical device review program. They provide FDA with more resources to maintain the cutting-edge scientific expertise necessary to provide timely review and ensure the safety of the increasingly complex devices coming to market. Patients and practitioners, in turn, will have access to safe and effective medical devices more quickly.

This law contains certain exemptions from user fees. It exempts any application for a device intended solely for pediatric use. It should be noted that changing the intended use from pediatric use to adult use requires a new submission, which would be subject to the review fee at the time of submission. Any application from a state or federal government entity is also exempt from user fees so long as the device is not to be distributed commercially. A 510(k) submission received from a third-party reviewer,

Table 5.4 FY 2010 device review user fees (U.S. dollars).

Application	Standard fee	SB < $1M
510(k)	$4,007	$2,004
513(g)	$2,941	$1,470
Premarket application (PMA, PDP, Biologics License Application [BLA], Postmarketing Requirement [PMR])	$217,787	$54,447
First premarket application from firms with gross receipts or sales ≤ $30 million	N/A	Waived
Panel-track supplement	$163,340	$40,845
Efficacy supplement (for BLA)	$217,787	$54,447
180-day supplement	$32,668	$8,167
Real-time supplement	$15,245	$3,811
30-day notice	$3,485	$1,742
Annual fee for periodic reporting on a Class III device	$7,623	$1,906

as discussed below in part 2, Premarket Notification (510[k]), is exempt from the user fee; however, the third party does charge the submitter a fee for its review.

The user fee program is described in detail on the FDA website at:

http://www.fda.gov/MedicalDevices/DeviceRegulationand
Guidance/Overview/MedicalDeviceUserFeeandModernization
ActMDUFMA/default.htm

and

http://www.fda.gov/MedicalDevices/DeviceRegulation
andGuidance/GuidanceDocuments/ucm089753.htm

Section 11. CDRH Premarket Review Submission Cover Sheet

FDA recommends that each premarket review submission be accompanied by a completed Premarket Review Submission Cover Sheet, FDA Form 3514. This cover sheet is applicable to all device premarket-type submissions including:

- PMA/PDP/HDEs and their supplements

- 510(k)s

- IDEs

- Class II and Class III exemption petitions

- 513(g) inquiries

- Pre-submission meetings

The completion of a Premarket Review Submission Cover Sheet is voluntary and will not affect any Food and Drug Administration decision concerning the submission, but it will help FDA's Center for Devices and Radiological Health process the submission more efficiently by placing administrative data elements in a consistent format for data entry purposes. The cover sheet was developed to reduce the number of administrative deficiencies common in many submissions. It can be found at:

http://www.fda.gov/downloads/AboutFDA/ReportsManuals
Forms/Forms/UCM080872.pdf

PART 2. PREMARKET NOTIFICATION (510[k])

Section 1. Background

Legislative Scheme for Marketing Applications

Prior to May 28, 1976, medical devices, per se, were not regulated as an entity. Some products that are now medical devices were regulated as new drugs and required an approved New Drug Application.

On May 28, 1976, the Medical Device Amendments of 1976 (MDA) amended the Federal Food, Drug, and Cosmetic Act (FDCA) for the purpose of directly regulating medical devices. Medical devices thus became regulated under the FDCA.

Under the MDA, a manufacturer must submit a premarket notification (510[k]) to FDA at least 90 days prior to introducing a medical device into commercial distribution unless it is the subject of an approved PMA or otherwise exempt from 510(k).

Purpose of the 510(k) Program

The primary purpose of the 510(k) program is to provide to FDA the opportunity to review a device before it is placed into commercial distribution. The essence of this review is to determine whether a device does not require a PMA because it is substantially equivalent (SE) to a predicate device identified in the 510(k). If the device is found to be SE, the manufacturer may proceed to marketing. If the device is found to be not substantially equivalent (NSE), the manufacturer will have to submit a PMA before marketing the device. Thus, the 510(k) review will identify new devices that must be placed automatically into Class III and undergo premarket approval or reclassification before they can be marketed. Some have argued that the 510(k) program is, in fact, a classification procedure because an NSE new device is in Class III and an SE new device is in the same regulatory class as the device to which it is found equivalent.

FDA provides a 510(k) home page at:

http://www.fda.gov/MedicalDevices/DeviceRegulationand
Guidance/HowtoMarketYourDevice/PremarketSubmissions/
PremarketNotification510k/default.htm

Section 2. Applicability

Devices Covered by 510(k)

Unless exempted by statute or regulation, the requirements of Section 510(k) apply to all Class I and Class II devices and a few Class III devices. The kinds of devices that are not covered by 510(k) include:

- Pre-amendment devices

- Unfinished devices

- Finished devices not sold in the United States

- Devices covered under another 510(k), for example, a private-labeled device being manufactured or distributed by a third party licensed by the 510(k) holder

- Custom devices

- General purpose articles

- Veterinary devices

Exempted Devices

FDA has exempted from 510(k) most Class I devices and many Class II devices. In determining whether a 510(k) is required for any particular device, it is important to confirm the exempt status. Exemption of devices is discussed in Chapter 1, part 13, section 4, Classification of Medical Devices.

Persons Covered by 510(k)

There are a variety of persons involved in the development, manufacture, and marketing of medical devices. These include manufacturers, importers, distributors, and relabelers. Some manufacturers develop their own devices while other manufacturers are merely contract manufacturers and do not market the devices they make for others. Distributors only buy and resell medical devices within the distribution chain and do not affect the manufacturing or labeling of the device.

In general, manufacturers wishing to introduce a device into the U.S. market must submit a 510(k) for review by FDA. However, it is important to distinguish between different types of manufacturers. Some types of manufacturers have to submit 510(k)s while other types do not depending on the functions they perform and the nature and intended use of the device, as explained below:

- An important factor in determining who has to submit a 510(k) relates to who has developed the specifications for the device. If a manufacturer develops its own specifications for the device and makes the finished product for marketing in the United States, it must submit a 510(k) for marketing clearance.

- If a manufacturer makes a finished device under contract for another person who has developed the specifications and who will be marketing the device in the United States, the manufacturer does not need to submit a 510(k). In this case, the specification developer is the one who would submit the 510(k), not the contract manufacturer. Thus, a contract manufacturer that manufactures a device under contract according to someone else's specifications is not required to submit a 510(k).

- A manufacturer of an accessory to a finished device that is sold to the end user must submit a 510(k) prior to marketing the accessory. An accessory is a device product that is used in conjunction with another device.

- A manufacturer of a device component is not required to submit a 510(k) unless the component is promoted for sale to an end user as a replacement part.

- A foreign manufacturer or foreign exporter that imports a medical device for sale in the United States, or the U.S. representative of the foreign manufacturer/exporter introducing a device into the U.S. market must submit a 510(k) for premarket clearance.

Repackagers or relabelers may be required to submit a 510(k) if they significantly change the labeling or otherwise affect any condition of the device. Significant labeling changes might include modification of manuals, such as adding a new intended use, deleting or adding warnings or contraindications, and so on. Operations such as sterilization could alter the condition of the device. However, most repackagers or relabelers who only add their company names and wording such as "Distributed by _____" or "Manufactured for _____" are not required to submit a 510(k).

A distributor or importer who furthers the marketing of a device and does not alter labeling or change the device does not require a 510(k) because the manufacturer or foreign exporter has to obtain the 510(k) clearance.

Section 3. Types of 510(k)s

An applicant may choose from three types of 510(k) submissions for marketing clearance: a traditional, a special, or an abbreviated 510(k).

Traditional 510(k)

A traditional 510(k) is one that is not a special or abbreviated 510(k). For a discussion of the form and content of a 510(k), see section 4 below.

Special 510(k)

A manufacturer may submit a "Special 510(k): Device Modification" for a modification to a device that has been cleared under the 510(k) process. The Special 510(k) allows the manufacturer to declare conformance to design controls without providing the data. While the basic content requirements of the 510(k) remain the same, this type of submission would also reference the cleared 510(k) number and contain a "Declaration of Conformity" with design control requirements.

Abbreviated 510(k)

A manufacturer may submit an abbreviated 510(k), which relies on the use of guidance documents, special controls, and recognized standards. An abbreviated 510(k) submission must include the elements required in a traditional premarket notification. Under certain conditions, it may not be necessary to submit test data in an abbreviated 510(k). Device manufacturers may choose to submit an abbreviated 510(k) when:

- A guidance document exists
- A special control has been established, or
- FDA has recognized a relevant consensus standard

In an abbreviated 510(k) submission, manufacturers elect to provide summary reports on the use of guidance documents or special controls or declarations of conformity to recognized standards to expedite the review of a submission. This saves the need to provide detailed data and information that is covered by these reference documents. It should be noted, however, that FDA reserves the right to verify the existence of the data necessary to support compliance with these guidances and standards.

510(k) Paradigm

FDA has issued a guidance document that contains detailed information on selecting the right kind of 510(k) to submit. The guidance contains a flowchart that is a graphical depiction of how to determine which type of the aforementioned 510(k)s is appropriate for a particular device. This paradigm is presented at:

> http://www.fda.gov/MedicalDevices/DeviceRegulationand
> Guidance/GuidanceDocuments/ucm080187.htm

Section 4. The 510(k) and Substantial Equivalence

Format of a 510(k)

A 510(k) technically is a "notification" and is different than most other types of FDA premarket applications. There is no official 510(k) "form" to complete. FDA does recommend, however, that the 510(k) be accompanied by the CDRH Premarket Review Submission Cover Sheet, Form 3514, as discussed in part 1, section 12 above.

Since a 510(k) is used to demonstrate that a new device is substantially equivalent to a predicate device, it must provide a comparison between the device to be marketed and the predicate device or devices. Even though there is no official form for a 510(k), each 510(k) must comply with the following:

- Specify the appropriate address for CDRH, CBER, or CDER
- Be bound into a volume or volumes, where necessary
- Be submitted in duplicate on standard size paper, including the original and two copies of the cover letter
- Be submitted separately for each product the manufacturer intends to market
- Designate "510(k) Notification" in the cover letter

Content of a 510(k)—Basic Information

A 510(k) must contain certain descriptive and performance data and information, as necessary, to demonstrate SE, as well as other important information. The 510(k) should include:

- The generic, brand, and classification name of the device
- The establishment registration number, if applicable
- The class of the device, or why the class is not included
- Labels, labeling, and advertisements to describe the device, the intended use, and directions for use
- Substantial equivalence data and information
- A discussion of modifications of the device that might affect the safety or effectiveness
- A discussion of new or different indications for use
- A 510(k) Summary or 510(k) Statement

- A Truthful and Accuracy Statement, and

- A Class III Certification, if necessary

Determination of Substantial Equivalence

The purpose of a 510(k) is to demonstrate that the device to be marketed is at least as safe and effective, that is, substantially equivalent, to a legally marketed device that is not subject to the PMA requirements. Submitters must compare their device to one or more legally marketed devices and make and support their substantial equivalency claims.

To further clarify the meaning of "substantial equivalence" Congress provided the following guidance on substantial equivalence in the *Report by the Committee on Interstate and Foreign Commerce,* H.R. Rep. No. 94-853, at pages 36–37:

> The term "substantially equivalent" is not intended to be so narrow as to refer only to devices that are identical to marketed devices nor so broad as to refer to devices which are intended to be used for the same purposes as marketed products. The committee believes that the term should be construed narrowly where necessary to assure the safety and effectiveness of a device but not narrowly where differences between a new device and a marketed device do not relate to safety and effectiveness. Thus, differences between "new" and marketed devices in materials, design, or energy source, for example, would have a bearing on the adequacy of information as to a new device's safety and effectiveness, and such devices should be automatically classified into Class III. On the other hand, copies of devices marketed prior to enactment, or devices whose variations are immaterial to safety and effectiveness would not necessarily fall under the automatic classification scheme.

This has been interpreted by FDA to mean that a claim of substantial equivalence does not mean the new and predicate devices must be identical. Substantial equivalence is established with respect to the device's intended use, design, energy used or delivered, materials, chemical composition, manufacturing process, performance, safety, effectiveness, labeling, biocompatibility, standards, and other characteristics, as applicable.

Thus, a device is substantially equivalent to a predicate device if, in comparison to the predicate, it has (1) the same intended use as the predicate and (2) the same technological characteristics as the predicate. A device may also be found to be SE if the device under review has the same intended use as the predicate and has different technological characteristics but, based on the information submitted to FDA, it (1) does not raise new questions of safety and effectiveness and (2) demonstrates that the device is at least as safe and effective as the legally marketed device.

FDA's decision to find a device SE entails a complex decision-making process. This process is described in detail in the guidance document "510(k) Submission Process," which appears at:

http://www.fda.gov/MedicalDevices/DeviceRegulationand Guidance/HowtoMarketYourDevice/PremarketSubmissions/ PremarketNotification510k/ucm070201.htm

As a further aid in making the SE determination and to bring transparency to the process, FDA has published the documents that are used by FDA reviewers in making an SE determination. The "510(k) Review Template" can be found at:

http://www.fda.gov/MedicalDevices/DeviceRegulationand Guidance/HowtoMarketYourDevice/PremarketSubmissions/ PremarketNotification510k/ucm071420.htm

The substantive decisions that are made during the review are best understood from the SE decision-making flowchart "510(k) 'Substantial Equivalence' Decision Making Process," which provides a graphic description of the steps in this process and which can be found on the FDA website at:

http://www.fda.gov/MedicalDevices/DeviceRegulationand Guidance/HowtoMarketYourDevice/PremarketSubmissions/ PremarketNotification510k/ucm134783.htm

Data Requirements

The primary data that are used in making a determination of SE consist of nonclinical data. Only about 10 to 15 percent of 510(k)s require clinical data. This is due to the nature of devices and the questions that have to be answered related to substantial equivalence. A great deal of the supporting data used to show equivalence is of a comparative and descriptive nature particularly susceptible to nonclinical laboratory testing. As stated above, the data would relate to a comparison of each device's intended use, design, energy used or delivered, materials, chemical composition, manufacturing process, performance, biocompatibility, conformance to standards, and labeling. Examples of the kinds of tests that might be used include stressing to failure, simulating long-term performance, and evaluating histopathological responses. The argument for this approach is that if the devices are similar enough in their characteristics and test results, the devices should both be of the same general level of safety and effectiveness.

There are times, however, when there is a need for a clinical study. This could be dictated by the degree of difference between the subject device and the predicate based on differences in design or new indications for use. Perhaps the bench and animal testing are unable to answer all of the questions raised. Other 510(k)s for certain devices, for example, non-invasive blood pressure machines, always require clinical data.

The types of clinical studies may differ depending on the device and the questions that need to be answered. 510(k) clinical studies are generally, but not always, confirmatory in nature and may be used to prove the validity of the concept of the device. Confirmatory studies usually require only a small sample size with a single arm that is historically controlled. Sometimes peer-reviewed literature articles may suffice. Then again, if the issues are more complex, a more traditional clinical study may be needed.

510(k) Statement

A 510(k) Statement is a statement asserting that all information in a premarket notification submission regarding safety and effectiveness will be made available within 30 days of a request by any person if the device described in the premarket notification submission is determined to be substantially equivalent. The information to be made available will be a duplicate of the premarket notification submission, including any adverse safety and effectiveness information, but excluding all patient identifiers and trade secret or confidential commercial information.

510(k) Summary

A 510(k) Summary is a separate section of the submission. It contains sufficient detail to provide an understanding of the basis for a determination of substantial equivalence. The 510(k) Summary is important to FDA and the Summary must contain the following information:

- The basis or rationale for substantial equivalence

- The submitter's name, address, and contact person

- The generic, brand, and classification name of the device

- An identification of a predicate device

- A description of the device similar to that found in the labeling or promotional materials, including:

  - Its functions

– The scientific concepts

– Any significant physical characteristics and performance characteristics (design, materials, properties)

– A statement of the intended uses of the device

– The diseases and conditions to be treated, and

– The patient population to be served

If the 510(k) is based on an assessment of performance data, then it must include a discussion of:

• The nonclinical tests referenced or relied on

• The clinical tests (patients, safety and effectiveness outcomes, adverse events, and so on), and

• The conclusions drawn from the testing

Upon clearance of the 510(k), the 510(k) summary is posted on the FDA website in the 510(k) database at:

http://www.fda.gov/MedicalDevices/ProductsandMedical
Procedures/DeviceApprovalsandClearances/510kClearances/
ucm089319.htm

The search screen for this database can be found at:

http://www.accessdata.fda.gov/scripts/cdrh/cfdocs/cfPMN/
pmn.cfm

Truthful and Accuracy Certification

This is a statement that the submitter believes, to the best of his or her knowledge, that all data and information submitted in the premarket notification are truthful and accurate and that no material fact has been omitted. This requirement is imposed so that there is an individual who takes personal responsibility for the accuracy and completeness of the submission.

Class III Certification

FDA regulations require, at 21 CFR 807.94, a 510(k) to contain the following statement when claiming substantial equivalence to certain devices classified into Class III:

(a) A Class III certification submitted as part of a premarket notification shall state as follows:

I certify, in my capacity as (position held in company), of (company name), that I have conducted a reasonable search of all information known or otherwise available about the types and causes of safety or effectiveness problems that have been reported for the (type of device). I further certify that I am aware of the types of problems to which the (type of device) is susceptible and that, to the best of my knowledge, the following summary of the types and causes of safety or effectiveness problems about the (type of device) is complete and accurate.

(b) The statement in paragraph (a) of this section should be signed by the certifier, clearly identified as "class III certification," and included at the beginning of the section of the premarket notification submission that sets forth the Class III summary.

Section 5. FDA Action on a 510(k)

After review of a premarket notification, FDA will take one of the following actions:

1. Issue an order declaring the device to be substantially equivalent (SE) to a legally marketed predicate device.

2. Issue an order declaring the device to be not substantially equivalent (NSE) to any legally marketed predicate device. This would mean a PMA is required for marketing approval.

3. Send a request for additional information (AI) letter.

4. Withhold the decision until a certification or financial disclosure statement is submitted to FDA.

5. Advise the applicant that a premarket notification is not required.

When FDA finds the device to be SE, the decision is referred to as "clearance" as opposed to "approval."

FDA's Decision-Making Process

The FDA decision-making process on a 510(k) begins with the completion of the "Screening Checklist for Traditional/Abbreviated Premarket Notification [510(k)] Submissions." The purpose of the checklist is to determine whether all of the necessary elements are present in the 510(k) so a full and complete review can be made. This checklist can be found on the FDA website at:

http://www.fda.gov/MedicalDevices/DeviceRegulationand
Guidance/HowtoMarketYourDevice/PremarketSubmissions/
PremarketNotification510k/ucm071360.htm

Once a complete 510(k) is received, FDA will review the 510(k) to determine whether the device is SE. The SE determination is discussed above under the topics "Determination of Substantial Equivalence" and "Data Requirements."

Third-Party Reviews

In order to expedite the processing of 510(k)s, FDA has an "Accredited Persons Program" that allows third parties to review 510(k)s. Under this program, FDA has accredited third parties that are authorized to conduct the primary review of 510(k)s for eligible devices. The devices eligible for third-party review can be found at:

http://www.accessdata.fda.gov/scripts/cdrh/cfdocs/cfThirdParty/
current.cfm

Persons who are required to submit 510(k)s for these devices may elect to contract with and submit a 510(k) directly to the third party. The accredited person conducts the primary review of the 510(k) and forwards its review, recommendation, and the 510(k) to FDA. FDA has a 30-day turnaround time in which to issue a final determination on the third-party recommendation. 510(k) submitters who do not wish to use an accredited person may submit their 510(k)s directly to FDA.

A list of accredited persons for third-party review can be found at:

http://www.accessdata.fda.gov/scripts/cdrh/cfdocs/cfthirdparty/
accredit.cfm

Confidentiality of Information

There are very specific confidentiality provisions related to 510(k)s. In broad and general terms, the FDA will disclose publicly the existence of a 510(k) when the device is on the market, that is, introduced or delivered for introduction into interstate commerce for commercial distribution, or when the person submitting the premarket notification submission has disclosed, through advertising or any other manner, his intent to market the device to scientists, market analysts, exporters, or other individuals who are not in a confidential relationship with the manufacturer. All of the nuances of these provisions can be found at:

http://www.accessdata.fda.gov/scripts/cdrh/cfdocs/cfcfr/
CFRSearch.cfm

In any case, within 30 days of an SE letter, FDA will make the 510(k) Summary available.

Section 6. Marketing a 510(k) Device

Until the submitter receives an order declaring a 510(k) device SE, the submitter may not proceed to market the device. Once the device is determined to be SE, it can then be marketed in the United States. The SE determination is usually made within 90 FDA review days and is made based on the information submitted by the submitter. If FDA determines that a device is not substantially equivalent, the applicant may take any of the following actions:

- Resubmit another 510(k) with new data

- Request a Class I or Class II designation through the *de novo* process

- File a reclassification petition

- Submit a premarket approval application

The determination by FDA that a 510(k) device is SE is considered to be a "clearance" for marketing the device and does not denote official approval of the device. Any representation that creates an impression of "approval" of such a device by FDA is misleading and constitutes misbranding.

Section 7. Custom Device Exemption

Custom devices do not require a cleared 510(k) before shipment in interstate commerce. Custom devices are discussed in Chapter 1, part 13, section 9, Custom Devices.

Section 8. Request under Section 513(g) of the Act

If there is doubt about the regulatory status or class into which a device belongs, the party may submit a written request under Section 513(g) of the FDCA for a determination by FDA. The inquiry should provide a device description with the intended uses of the device and the draft labeling. The agency provides some guidance on the content of a 513(g) inquiry and some sample questions that would be appropriate for response by FDA:

- Is my product subject to FDA device requirements?

- Is my device exempt from the 510(k) requirements of the FDCA?

- Do I need a 510(k) for a modification to my legally marketed device?

- What is the least burdensome regulatory pathway for a device that introduces a new technology or a new intended use?

The agency has 60 days to provide a written statement of the classification of such device and the requirements applicable to the device. It should be noted that a response to a 513(g) is an opinion and not a clearance or approval to market the device.

Section 9. Upcoming 510(k) Program Changes

FDA has been evaluating its 510(k) submission and review program to determine how the 510(k) process can be improved. One part of this effort was the commissioning of the National Academy of Sciences' Institute of Medicine (IOM) to study the premarket notification program. The IOM, which is not part of the FDA, will be able to provide independent, objective, evidence-based advice about the program. The IOM will look into two principal questions:

- Does the current 510(k) process optimally protect patients and promote innovation in support of public health?

- If not, what legislative, regulatory, or administrative changes are recommended to achieve the goals of the 510(k) process?

The IOM study is not scheduled to be completed until the late spring or summer of 2011, but the agency is taking other steps in the meantime. These include:

- Creating an internal task force on the use of science in regulatory decision making

- Developing an effective compliance strategy

- Optimally integrating premarket and post-market information

- Increasing transparency in decision making

- Establishing clear procedures to resolve differences of opinion

FDA has also held public meetings to gather ideas and to exchange views on how to improve the 510(k) program.

This process of 510(k) program review may result in many changes in the program. The following list of possible changes is offered merely to illustrate the kinds of changes that may occur and should not be taken as predictive of future outcomes of this review process:

- Providing a clear and transparent process that will allow the agency to rescind a 510(k)

- Provide additional clarity regarding key concepts in the SE decision-making process as it relates to the indications for use or technological characteristics

- Putting limits on technological creep by limiting the use of outdated predicate devices or the number of SE devices that may be a predicate device

- Providing predictability to industry regarding the need for nonclinical and clinical evidence required to establish substantial equivalence

- Expanding the use of information external to the 510(k) submission and the labeling in determining the intended use of the device

As a result of all of this activity, CDRH issued two preliminary reports with findings and recommendations that will have an impact on the 510(k) program in particular and on the premarket review program in general. The two reports are:

- *CDRH Preliminary Internal Evaluations—Volume I: 510(k) Working Group Preliminary Report and Recommendations*

- *CDRH Preliminary Internal Evaluations—Volume II: Task Force on the Utilization of Science in Regulatory Decision Making Preliminary Report and Recommendations.*

The first report, volume I, contains nine individual findings and recommendations related to a variety of topics of importance to the 510(k) program. Examples of the types of actions these proposals may elicit include clarifying the meanings of "substantial equivalence," "same intended use," "indications for use," and "different questions of safety and effectiveness." Other recommendations relate to improving guidance to industry, establishing a new class (IIb), additional training for FDA staff, and improving the availability of device information.

The second report, volume II, has six findings and recommendations related to the acquisition, dissemination, and use of scientific information related to device evaluation.

These reports have been issued by CDRH for public review and comment. The full reports are available at the following web page and its internal links:

http://www.fda.gov/AboutFDA/CentersOffices/CDRH/
CDRHReports/ucm220272.htm

After the review period, FDA may take a variety of actions to implement these recommendations, including new policies, procedures, and regulations. This process will play out over the next year or two. It will be important for professionals in the medical device field to maintain their vigilance, follow events in the trade press and their professional journals, and monitor the FDA website to learn what changes are made and to determine how they might affect their practice.

PART 3. PMAs/PDPs/HDEs

The premarket approval application (PMA), product development protocol (PDP), and the humanitarian device exemption (HDE) are true premarket approval applications requiring review and approval by FDA. They are, in effect, a private license granted to the applicant for marketing a particular medical device.

The PMA and PDP are reviewed by FDA to determine whether there is sufficient valid scientific evidence to provide a reasonable assurance of the safety and effectiveness (S&E) of the device for its intended use under the conditions of use expressed in the labeling.

The HDE has some special considerations that are discussed in section 10 below.

The "S&E" acronym for safety and effectiveness of a PMA device should be distinguished from the "SE," or substantial equivalence, required for clearance of a 510(k) device.

The FDA's PMA home page can be found at:

http://www.fda.gov/MedicalDevices/DeviceRegulationand
Guidance/HowtoMarketYourDevice/PremarketSubmissions/
PremarketApprovalPMA/default.htm

Section 1. PMA Overview

Devices Covered by Premarket Approval (PMA) Application

As discussed in Chapter 1, part 13, section 4, Classification of Medical Devices, Class III devices are those devices that support or sustain human life, are of substantial importance in preventing impairment of human health, or that present a potential, unreasonable risk of illness or injury. Due to the level of risk associated with Class III devices, general and special controls alone are insufficient to assure the safety and effectiveness of Class III devices. Accordingly, Class III devices require an approved PMA (or the alternative PDP or HDE, as discussed in sections below) in order to be commercially distributed in interstate commerce in the United States.

There are, however, some Class III devices that may be shipped in interstate commerce without an approved PMA. The following are examples of types of devices that could be in Class III but may be shipped without an approved PMA because they are covered by other authorities or requirements:

- Investigational device

- Custom device

- Research device

- Components

- A device reclassified as Class I or II

- A transitional device that is marketed under a valid NDA or Abbreviated New Drug Application (ANDA) as a drug or antibiotic for which FDA has not called for a PMA

- Class III pre-amendment device for which FDA has not called for a PMA

Types of PMA Submissions

There are three types of PMA submissions that must be considered:

- Original PMA

- PMA amendment

- PMA supplement

An original PMA is required for a new device that is not substantially equivalent. Whether a device is substantially equivalent is discussed above in part 2, section 4, The 510(k) and Substantial Equivalence. An original PMA may also be required when there are changes to an existing device that is not the subject of the original PMA and the modifications result in a new device.

A PMA amendment may be required for the submission of data or information that is necessary before a final FDA action is rendered on a pending original PMA or pending PMA supplement.

A PMA supplement would be the appropriate application for changes to a device, its labeling, or manufacture after final FDA action on an original PMA or a previously approved PMA supplement.

Section 2. Original PMA Submissions

An original PMA application may be either a traditional or modular PMA. A *traditional* PMA is merely a PMA submitted as a full and complete document with all of the necessary sections included.

A *modular* PMA is one that is submitted in discrete sections as they become available. Separate sections may be submitted at different times for the nonclinical test data, manufacturing information, and clinical trial results. For example, a clinical trial may be ongoing for several years, but the nonclinical data or manufacturing data may be complete. The completed data and information may be submitted in individual modules for review and acceptance by FDA. In order to use the modular submission, the applicant must first obtain FDA agreement with this approach.

Section 3. Format and Content of a PMA Submission

A PMA is a large, complex, and comprehensive document. The purpose of a PMA is to establish reasonable assurance of the safety and effectiveness of the device for the intended use in the identified patient population. The data and information provided for this purpose must constitute valid scientific evidence. This evidence will usually consist of design information, nonclinical test data, and the results of clinical studies, all of which have been discussed in detail in previous chapters of the book.

General Instructions/Advice

Although not technically part of the format or content of a PMA, there are certain things external to the PMA an applicant can do to help expedite the review of a PMA. For example:

- Request pre-PMA meetings. FDA encourages this as a means to avoid confusion and misunderstandings at a later time.

- Call FDA if there are any questions, but save the phone calls and meeting requests for when they are really necessary. Avoid excessive calls to check on the status of the review. Constant interruptions will only divert the attention of a reviewer from the actual review of applications.

- Make sure the official contact person identified in the submission is someone who is readily available. If not, it will only create delays in the review of the application. Also, it is beneficial and can save time when subject experts can speak to each other directly.

- Be prepared for quick turnaround times. Keep commitments on sending in additional information, but don't sacrifice quality for speed.

- When deficiencies are received, ask for clarification, if needed. This will help avoid inappropriate or incorrect responses that will cause delays and duplicative work. If deficiencies are not appropriate, contact the lead reviewer and the branch chief.

- Ensure that the manufacturing sites are ready to be inspected.

- Have all documentation readily available to validate the accuracy and completeness of the data and information in the PMA.

PMA Cover Letter

FDA recommends the format shown in Figure 5.1 for cover letters to accompany each original PMA.

PMA Cover Sheet

See part 1, section 12 above.

PMA Summary

Every PMA must contain a summary of the PMA. The summary in a PMA is similar to the summary in a 510(k) and serves the same general purpose. It provides an overview of the contents of the submission and the data, and the theory on which a determination of safety and effectiveness can be based. The reviewer then has a concise statement of the critical information in the submission. The PMA summary must contain the following information:

- The indications for use

- A description of the device

- Alternative practices and procedures

[Date]

Document Mail Center (HFZ-401)
Center for Devices and Radiological Health
Food and Drug Administration
9200 Corporate Blvd.
Rockville, MD 20850

Subject: Original PMA for [device trade name and model number, if applicable]

To whom it may concern:

[Applicant's name] is submitting this original premarket approval application for the [device trade name], [device generic name] intended for use in [indication for use].

Clinical studies of the above device were initiated on [date] and [were/were not] conducted under an approved investigational device exemption [give IDE number if a significant-risk device]. [If applicable, include the FDA reference number for any premarket notification, reclassification petition, or color additive petition submitted for this device.]

[Include a paragraph providing the name and address of each facility involved in the manufacture of the device, and indicate whether the facility is prepared for an FDA inspection. If not prepared, provide an expected date when the facility will be ready for inspection. If a waiver of the QS information is requested, provide an anticipated date that the information will be provided.]

[If another document is incorporated by reference, for example, a master file, please include the original letter of authorization as an attachment to this cover letter.]

The existence of this PMA and the data and other information that it contains are confidential, and the protection afforded to such confidential information by 18 USC 1905, 21 USC 331(j), 5 USC 552, and other applicable laws is hereby claimed. [Tip: confidentiality claims can not be made unless the applicant has complied with the applicable requirements.]

If there are questions regarding this submission, [name] may be contacted at [give telephone number including area code].

Sincerely yours,

[Signature]

[Name and title of applicant's representative]

Figure 5.1 FDA-recommended PMA cover letter.

- Marketing history
- A summary of studies that includes:
  - A summary of the nonclinical laboratory studies submitted in the application
  - A summary of the clinical investigations submitted in the application
  - The conclusions drawn from the studies

The information provided should apply only to a single accompanying submission. The cover sheet for an amendment or supplement should identify the document number and type of submission, and then provide only the information that has changed. An example of a PMA cover sheet, for the Independence iBOT 3000 Mobility System, can be seen on the FDA website at:

http://www.fda.gov/ohrms/dockets/ac/02/briefing/3910b1_08_
summary%20data.doc

Content of a PMA

In addition to the PMA summary, the regulations identify other required components of a PMA. Aside from the following list of elements that are required in the PMA, it is useful to consider providing some general comments about the preparation of the PMA. Preparing the PMA will require significant planning and time to write, so it is important to start early in the device development process. The text must be in English, and it will receive great scrutiny by FDA.

It is important to ensure that the submission is well organized, with a table of contents, separate sections, and full pagination. There should be consistency throughout the submission. Respective sections are reviewed by different types of reviewers, so it is important to carefully consider the audience.

All text, tables, and graphs should be clearly labeled and legible. In providing substantive information, there should be no data dumps. Also, no test reports should be omitted unless FDA has agreed.

The following major elements are expressly required in a PMA:

- The name and address of the applicant
- A detailed table of contents
- An executive summary, as discussed above

- A complete description of the device, including pictorial representations

- References to any performance standards relevant to the safety or effectiveness of the device

- A section for nonclinical studies

- A section containing the results of clinical investigations

- A bibliography of all published reports, whether adverse or supportive, that concern the safety or effectiveness of the device

- An environmental assessment

- A financial certification or disclosure

In addition to the original PMA submission, periodic reports updating the S&E information are required. This requires the applicant to keep FDA informed on recent developments concerning the device that transpired after submission of the PMA.

Another requirement that was adopted after the promulgation of the PMA regulation is the certification that the clinical study was registered with NIH in the national Clinical Trials Data Bank, which is discussed in Chapter 4, part 8, National Clinical Trials Data Bank.

Device Description

Describing a device involves describing the characteristics of the device and each of the functional components or ingredients of the device if the device consists of more than one physical component or ingredient. It would include an explanation of how the device functions, the basic scientific concepts and principles of operation that form the basis for the device, and the significant physical and performance characteristics of the device. The properties of the device relevant to the diagnosis, treatment, prevention, cure, or mitigation of a disease or condition in the intended patient population would be important.

A brief description of the manufacturing process should be included if it will significantly enhance the reviewer's understanding of the device. The description should also include an analysis of the design, a failure mode and effects analysis (FMEA), and hazard analysis.

The generic name of the device, as well as any proprietary name or trade name, should be included along with pictures, drawings, or graphical representations of the device.

A further discussion of describing a device appears in Chapter 3, part 1, section 3, Device Description.

Nonclinical Laboratory Studies

The section of the PMA dealing with nonclinical studies should contain an introduction that provides the context and overview of respective subsections dealing with the specific tests that were conducted, including microbiological, toxicological, immunological, biocompatibility, stress, wear, shelf life, and other laboratory or animal tests as appropriate. It should set forth the background and the chronology for the testing. A general discussion of nonclinical laboratory studies can be found in Chapter 3, Nonclinical Testing and GLPs. The introduction should provide context with respect to design requirements, design controls, and design risk analysis. Also, see Chapter 2, Medical Device Design.

Beyond the introductory material, the subsection for each test should include a description of the objective of the study, a description of the experimental design of the study, a description of how the data were collected and analyzed, and a description of the results, whether positive, negative, or inconclusive. For each test, the test procedure or protocol should be included. The protocol for each test should contain the following information:

- The objective of the test and what the test is intended to accomplish.

- The rationale of why the test is appropriate.

- A description of the test setup.

- A diagram of the test setup.

- Identification of the test equipment used.

- The location of measurement instruments.

- A description of test conditions with rationale of how they relate to the anticipated clinical use.

- The sample size and the rationale for it.

- The data to be collected.

- The duration of the test and its rationale.

- The acceptance criteria and a justification as to why the acceptance criteria are suitable and how they relate to the device specification.

- An identification of the hardware and software version used.

- An identification of the differences between the device tested (for example, prototype, different models of the same device) and the device to be marketed, with an explanation of why the differences do not affect the outcome.

- If the protocol refers to other company documents, provide the documents.

There are two strategies for the presentation of the actual test data. The first approach would be to provide summaries for each test with references to the attached test reports. The second method is to provide detailed discussions of each test along with the test data, in which case there would be no need for attachments. These subsections should provide an analysis of the data and ensure that the test results meet the acceptance criteria.

Clinical Studies and Data

In dealing with the PMA section on clinical studies and clinical data, it is important to first distinguish whether or not the clinical trials were conducted under an approved IDE. FDA requests that this information be included in the cover letter depicted above so that the reviewer will have this information at the outset. This information is important because all of the clinical information collected pursuant to an IDE will be measured against the requirements of the IDE. Therefore, the PMA must identify any investigation conducted under an IDE, including the IDE number.

In effect, an applicable IDE will be merged with the PMA. This can be a significant benefit to the applicant because the clinical studies that were approved under the IDE will be acceptable if they were conducted in accordance with the IDE. On the other hand, a clinical study that was not the subject of an IDE, for example, an NSR study that was reviewed by an IRB, runs the risk of being found not acceptable when presented in the PMA for the first time.

For a PMA supported solely by data from one investigation, there should be a justification that shows that the data and other information from the single investigator are sufficient to demonstrate the safety and effectiveness of the device. It must also explain why and how the reproducibility of the study will be ensured.

The clinical section should include the following items:

- The clinical protocols

- A description of the device's clinical utility

- The indication for use and the study's hypothesis

- The number of investigators and the subjects per investigator

- Subject selection and exclusion criteria

- The study population, including demographics

- The study period or duration

- The study end points

- The safety and effectiveness data

- All adverse reactions and complications

- All patient discontinuation and patient complaints

- All device failures and replacements

- Tabulations of data from all individual subject report forms, and copies of such forms for each subject who died during a clinical investigation or who did not complete the investigation

- Statistical analyses of the clinical investigations, methods and results, and device failures and replacements

- Conclusions, from a clinical perspective

- Contraindications and precautions for use of the device

- Any other appropriate information from the clinical investigations

The PMA must account for all of the patients in the study and the outcomes achieved. See, for example, Figure 5.2 and Figure 5.3.

The statistical analysis plan should not be changed without prior consultation with FDA. Changes in the control group, changing from concurrent control to historical controls, crossover of control patients, changing the anticipated effect size to decrease the sample size, and increasing the sample size are examples of the kinds of changes that can lead to unintended ramifications that will be of concern to FDA.

Adverse event reporting is very important. The PMA should be consistent in how anticipated and unanticipated adverse events are categorized. It should avoid "cascading" events, and extremes in "lumping" and "splitting." It is important to work with FDA, during the IDE stage or before the trial begins, on how adverse events are to be categorized and reported on the case report forms.

Using a subgroup analysis to demonstrate safety or effectiveness for a device will raise issues and questions. Subgroup analyses are useful for

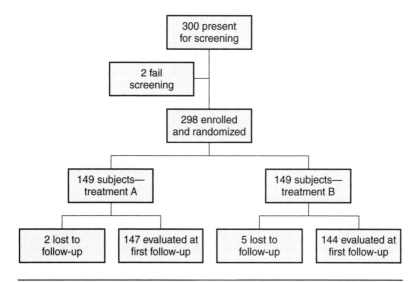

Figure 5.2 Hypothetical subject accountability chart.

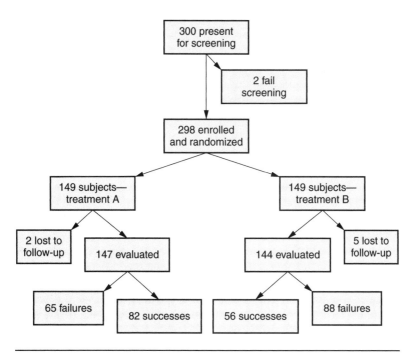

Figure 5.3 Hypothetical study outcome chart.

defining a particular group that benefited more or less than the overall patient population, but subgroup analyses are not generally acceptable to demonstrate S&E. They may be useful provided that an overall effect has been shown.

The PMA should address the "future concerns" items in IDE letters. The "future concerns" section of IDE letters contains information that FDA expects the sponsor to address in the PMA submission. It may include:

- Long-term biocompatibility or laboratory tests

- Labeling or indication limitations/issues

- Statistical issues

- Clinical trial design issues

Failure to address these concerns will raise questions and may lead to a delay in the review process.

The studies in the PMA should have been carefully monitored. If they were not, during the substantive review of the PMA or during a BIMO inspection questions might arise that could delay the review and approval process. Questions may have to be answered related to:

- Patient enrollment issues

- The application of the inclusion/exclusion criteria

- The adequacy of informed consent

- The reliability of the data collection and record keeping

- The completeness of adverse event reporting

- The use of agreed-on assessment tools or methods

- The integrity of the blinding process

- The accountability of those lost to follow-up

Regulatory Compliance Statements

The clinical study section should include a statement of compliance with certain related regulatory requirements. It should state whether each study was conducted in compliance with the Institutional Review Board and informed consent regulations and, if not, an explanation and the reasons for noncompliance. The same statement is required concerning the IDE regulation. These regulations are discussed in Chapter 4, Clinical Trials.

The information on nonclinical laboratory studies should include a statement that each such study was conducted in compliance with the Good

Laboratory Practice regulations, or, if the study was not conducted in compliance with such regulations, a brief statement of the reason for the noncompliance. See Chapter 3, part 2, Good Laboratory Practices.

A financial disclosure certification and financial disclosure statements must be included. See the discussion above in part 1, section 6, Financial Disclosure.

Manufacturing

The manufacturing section of the PMA must describe the methods used in, and the facilities and controls used for, the manufacture, processing, packing, storage, and, where appropriate, installation of the device, in sufficient detail so that a person generally familiar with current good manufacturing practices can make a knowledgeable judgment about the quality control used in the manufacture of the device. Manufacturing is discussed in detail in Chapter 7, Quality Systems and GMPs.

Labeling

The application should include all draft labeling, including an operator's manual, instructions for use, patient manual, promotional literature, and so on. The labeling is often the last part of the PMA that is resolved because the labeling can not be finalized until FDA knows all of the facts about the device and whether or not it is approvable. Some of the issues that are resolved in agreeing on the final labeling may include the prominent display in the labeling and in the advertising of warnings, hazards, or precautions important for the device's safe and effective use, including patient information, for example, information provided to the patient on alternative modes of therapy and on risks and benefits associated with the use of the device. Other aspects of labeling are discussed above in part 1, section 3, Labeling and Unapproved Uses.

Bibliography

A bibliography is an important part of a PMA because it may lead to information about a device and its prior use as a medical modality. It may lead to corroborating or impeaching information about the device. The bibliography should identify all published reports not submitted in the PMA, whether adverse or supportive, known to, or that should reasonably be known to, the applicant that concern the safety or effectiveness of the device.

The bibliography should identify, discuss, and analyze any other data, information, or report relevant to an evaluation of the safety and effectiveness of the device known to, or that should reasonably be known to, the applicant from any source, foreign or domestic, including information derived from investigations other than those proposed in the application, and from commercial marketing experience.

The PMA should include copies of such published reports or unpublished information in the possession of, or reasonably obtainable by, the applicant if an FDA advisory committee or FDA requests such copies.

Section 4. The Determination of Safety and Effectiveness and the Summary of Safety and Effectiveness Data

In making a determination on the approvability of a PMA, FDA will take into account the analysis and review memos prepared by the scientists on the review team and division managers, the recommendations of an advisory panel, and the results of preapproval BIMO and QSR inspections. Based on this lengthy and detailed evaluation, if the totality of evidence provides a reasonable assurance that a device is safe and effective for its intended use as set forth in the labeling, FDA will approve the PMA. If the assurance of safety and effectiveness is not present, FDA may deny approval of the PMA. As a last step in the approval or denial process, FDA will prepare and publish a Summary of Safety and Effectiveness Data (SSED) that will set forth the basis of the FDA decision.

Reasonable Assurances of Safety

During the evaluation of the data and information in a PMA, FDA will have to determine whether there is sufficient evidence of the safety of the device. There is a reasonable assurance that a device is safe when it can be determined, based on valid scientific evidence, *that the probable benefits to health outweigh any probable risks when it is:*

1. Used for its intended uses,

2. Under its intended conditions of use,

3. With adequate directions and warnings against unsafe use, and

4. The evidence demonstrates the absence of unreasonable risk of illness or injury when used as directed.

Reasonable Assurances of Effectiveness

Similarly, FDA will have to determine whether there is sufficient evidence in the PMA of the effectiveness of the device. There is a reasonable assurance that a device is effective when it can be determined, based on valid scientific evidence, *that its use will provide clinically significant results, in a significant portion of the target population, when it is*:

1. Used for its intended uses,

2. Used under its intended conditions of use,

3. With adequate directions and warnings against unsafe use.

Summary of Safety and Effectiveness Data

A Summary of Safety and Effectiveness Data (SSED) is a detailed summary of the safety and effectiveness data on which a PMA is approved or denied. The SSED is intended to present a reasoned, objective, and balanced critique of the scientific evidence that served as the basis of the decision to approve or deny the PMA. The SSED documents that there was a reasonable assurance of safety and effectiveness for the device as labeled based on the nonclinical and clinical studies described in the PMA. The SSED is a summation of both the positive and negative aspects of the PMA.

FDA is required to publish an SSED upon issuance of an order approving or denying the approval of a PMA. Originally, the SSED was prepared by FDA. Under current practices, the SSED is drafted by the applicant and submitted to FDA for review. This draft will be amended as necessary by FDA, and the SSED may go through an iterative process with the applicant before the SSED is finalized. Sometimes this process can take a substantial amount of time and work before the SSED is completed and published.

Approval or denial decisions for original PMA applications and panel-track supplements must include a detailed SSED. An abbreviated SSED is required for approval of a PMA based on a licensing agreement. The abbreviated SSED is acceptable because the scientific data on which the PMA relies were previously described in the SSED for the original PMA application that is being licensed.

Once the SSED is finalized, and upon approval of the PMA, FDA publishes all SSEDs on its website. An example of an SSED, for the CardioWest Temporary Total Artificial Heart, can be found at:

http://www.fda.gov/ohrms/dockets/dockets/04m0471/04m-0471-cr00001-02-SSED-vol42.pdf

As can be seen from this example, an SSED can be a lengthy and complex document. The FDA has posted more-detailed guidance on the preparation and content of a PMA, which includes information on the SSED, on its website at:

http://www.fda.gov/MedicalDevices/DeviceRegulationand
Guidance/HowtoMarketYourDevice/PremarketSubmissions/
PremarketApprovalPMA/ucm050289.htm

Section 5. PMA Meetings

There are several meetings between FDA and the applicant of a PMA that
are integral to the review process and the evaluation of a PMA. It behooves
the applicant to participate in these meetings so as to make the review process proceed as efficiently as possible.

Pre-PMA Submission Meeting

A pre-PMA meeting, as the name implies, takes place before a PMA is submitted to FDA. The purpose of this meeting is to allow the applicant the
opportunity to obtain input from FDA before submitting the application. It
is not an in-depth review but will allow the applicant to get guidance on the
specific application that will be submitted.

After scheduling the meeting, the applicant should provide FDA with a
pre-meeting package that includes:

- A description of the device and the proposed indication for use

- A brief summary of:

  - All pre-clinical tests

  - The clinical protocol and any protocol deviations or changes

  - The safety and effectiveness results, including patient
    accountability

- A description of:

  - Any changes to the statistical analysis plan

  - Any changes to the device since the IDE submission

During the meeting, the applicant should obtain FDA input on the desired
clinical data presentation for the PMA and on information regarding a
panel meeting and expedited review.

Day 100 Meeting

FDA, upon written request from the applicant, is required to meet with
the applicant no later than 100 days after the receipt and filing of a PMA
application unless the applicant agrees to another time. The purpose of the
meeting is to provide to the applicant an early preview of the review status

of the application. Prior to the meeting, FDA will inform the applicant in writing of any identified deficiencies and what information is required to correct those deficiencies. FDA must also promptly notify the applicant if it identifies additional deficiencies or any additional information required to complete agency review. The full FDA guidance for this type of meeting can be found at:

> http://www.fda.gov/MedicalDevices/DeviceRegulationand
> Guidance/GuidanceDocuments/ucm080190.htm

Other Meetings

Other meetings may occur at any time during the review of a PMA depending on the need to discuss and clarify issues that arise during review and upon the agreement of the sponsor and FDA.

Section 6. FDA Actions

Upon the receipt of a PMA, FDA will make various decisions and take various actions related to the PMA. The major FDA actions include:

- Filing or not filing the PMA
- Issuing a deficiency letter
- Issuing an approvable or not approvable letter
- Issuing an approval or denial of approval letter
- Adding conditions of approval to the approvable letter

A searchable list of PMA approvals, by year, can be found at:

> http://www.fda.gov/MedicalDevices/ProductsandMedical
> Procedures/DeviceApprovalsandClearances/PMAApprovals/
> ucm096300.htm

Section 7. PMA Conditions of Approval Requirements

Post-approval requirements are established in the PMA approval order. These are commonly referred to as "conditions of approval," which are mandatory under the regulations, as stated at 21 CFR 814.80:

> A device may not be manufactured, packaged, stored, labeled, distributed, or advertised in a manner that is inconsistent with any conditions to approval specified in the PMA approval order for the device.

The FDA may include any condition of approval it deems necessary to assure the continued safe and effective use of the device. The post-approval requirements that are discussed in this chapter are included below in the following sections: section 8, Post-Approval Reports, section 9, Adverse Reaction and Device Defect Reporting, and section 10, Post-Approval Studies.

FDA guidance on these requirements, "PMA Post-Approval Requirements," can be found at:

> http://www.fda.gov/MedicalDevices/DeviceRegulationand
> Guidance/HowtoMarketYourDevice/PremarketSubmissions/
> PremarketApprovalPMA/ucm050422.htm

There are several other types of post-approval requirements that must be considered. Some post-approval requirements are established through the promulgation of a regulation. These are discussed in Chapter 6, Post-Market Requirements, and include medical device reporting, post-market surveillance studies, medical device tracking, and recalls.

Section 8. Post-Approval Reports

An annual report is automatically required for an approved PMA, and it is included as a standing condition of approval in each PMA approval letter. The annual report has to be submitted at intervals of one year from the date of PMA approval. This report, and other post-approval reports that may be required in the PMA approval order, is an important tool that FDA relies on to gather information about the device during its aftermarket use in the healthcare setting. These reports give FDA a more complete picture of the post-market safety profile of the device.

Device Changes

Annual reports currently contain a variety of information, including information about manufacturing changes, design changes, and labeling changes that were made during the preceding year for the PMA product. The annual report must also contain an analysis of the reasons for the changes and indicate whether they were due to complaints, adverse events, or other reasons.

Under the requirement to report changes, when any significant chemical, physical, or other change or deterioration in the device, or any failure of the device to meet the specifications established in the approved PMA, are correctable by adjustments or other maintenance procedures described in the approved labeling, all such events known to the applicant must be included in the annual report unless specified otherwise in the conditions of approval to the PMA.

The annual report must also categorize these events and include the number of reported and otherwise known instances of each category during the reporting period. Additional information regarding these events should be submitted by the applicant when determined by FDA to be necessary to provide continued reasonable assurance of the safety and effectiveness of the device for its intended use.

Bibliography and Summary

In addition to the reporting of changes to the device, the annual report must also include a bibliography and summary of unpublished reports of data from any clinical or nonclinical study involving the device or a related device, and reports in the scientific literature concerning the device.

Device Changes Affecting S&E

After a PMA is approved, the PMA holder must submit a PMA supplement for any change to the device that affects the safety and effectiveness of the device. However, such changes may be included in the annual report, in lieu of a supplement, if FDA permits such reporting in the PMA approval letter or other correspondence for a specific device. Alternately, FDA may also permit such reporting for a generic type of device through an advisory opinion.

The reporting of such changes in the annual report relieves the manufacturer of the burden of submitting a PMA supplement and permits the manufacturer to make the change before reporting it to FDA. This also streamlines FDA's review of such changes that do not require a full review under a formal PMA supplement.

Other Changes

The other types of changes that must be reported in the annual report are certain changes that do not affect the safety and effectiveness of the device and would not require a PMA supplement. FDA may require specified changes of this nature to be reported to the agency in the annual report.

QSR/GMP Interface

It may be noted that many of the types of information required in post-approval reports are already part of the quality system practices of companies that comply with QSR regulations. For example, design controls already require the type of look-back and assessment that is expected as part of the annual report. Design controls are dealt with in Chapter 2, Medical Device Design, and the QSR regulations are covered in Chapter 7, Quality Systems and GMPs.

Section 9. Adverse Reaction and Device Defect Reporting

[*Note:* According to informal information from CDRH, PMA approval letters no longer automatically include adverse reaction and device defect reporting as a condition of approval. The following information is being provided because this change in policy has not been officially announced. However, it appears the agency will be relying on the Medical Device Reporting (MDR) regulation, discussed in Chapter 6, part 1, Medical Device Reporting, instead of the PMA approval letter for this type of information, which eliminates a previously existing and confusing duplication of requirements.]

FDA provides the following guidance in the guidance document "PMA Postapproval Requirements" cited above:

FDA has determined that in order to provide continued reasonable assurance of the safety and effectiveness of the device, the applicant shall submit an "Adverse Reaction Report" or "Device Defect Report," as applicable, within 10 days after the applicant receives or has knowledge of information concerning:

(1) A mix-up of the device or its labeling with another article.

(2) Any adverse reaction, side effect, injury, toxicity, or sensitivity reaction that is attributable to the device and

(a) has not been addressed by the device's labeling or

(b) has been addressed by the device's labeling, but is occurring with unexpected severity or frequency.

(3) Any significant chemical, physical, or other change or deterioration in the device or any failure of the device to meet the specifications established in the approved PMA that could not cause or contribute to death or serious injury but are not correctable by adjustments or other maintenance procedures described in the approved labeling. The report shall include a discussion of the applicant's assessment of the change, deterioration, or failure and any proposed or implemented corrective action by the applicant. When such events are correctable by adjustments or other maintenance procedures described in the approved labeling, all such events known to the applicant shall be included in the Annual Report described under "Postapproval Reports" above unless specified otherwise in the conditions of approval to this PMA. The post-approval report shall appropriately categorize these events and include the number of reported and otherwise known instances of each category during the reporting period. Additional

information regarding the events discussed above shall be submitted by the applicant when determined by FDA to be necessary to provide continued reasonable assurance of the safety and effectiveness of the device for its intended use.

If an adverse event and device defect report is required under a PMA approval order and is also reportable under the MDR regulation, the FDA advises that the event should be reported under the MDR program and listed in a PMA annual report with the notation that it is an MDR-reported event. This eliminates the need for duplicative reporting, which reduces the burden on the manufacturer and streamlines the FDA data management system.

Section 10. Post-Approval Studies

Devices are determined to be S&E at the time of approval. However, for certain devices the agency would like to review longer-term data dealing with specific concerns it may have with the device. When this occurs, FDA may include among the conditions of approval a requirement that the applicant conduct a long-term study to assure the continued safe and effective use of the device and to obtain the data and information desired. For example, long-term studies may include long-term IDE follow-up, maintenance of a patient registry, a clinical outcomes study, a pediatric study, fatigue testing, materials testing, device failure, a dosing study, and any type of study to produce the desired data.

In conducting a post-approval study (PAS), various protocols for varying periods of time are adopted depending on the device, risks presented, intended use, and patient population. The applicant will work with the CDRH Office of Surveillance and Biometrics (OSB), which has the lead review on the PAS.

The CDRH Post-Approval Studies Program encompasses design, tracking, oversight, and review responsibilities for studies mandated as a condition of approval of a PMA application, product development protocol (PDP) application, or humanitarian device exemption (HDE) application. The program helps ensure that well-designed post-approval studies are conducted effectively and efficiently and in the least burdensome manner.

OSB tracks all post-approval studies and maintains a publicly available web page to keep all stakeholders informed of the progress of each PAS. The web page displays general information regarding each PAS, as well as the overall study status (based on protocol-driven timelines and the adequacy of the data) and the applicant's reporting status for each submission due. The PAS database appears at:

http://www.accessdata.fda.gov/scripts/cdrh/cfdocs/cfPMA/pma_
pas.cfm

In addition to the post-approval studies required through the PMA process, the FDA is authorized to require a post-market surveillance study of any Class II or Class III device as specified in the regulations. These surveillance studies are discussed in Chapter 6, part 2, Post-Market Surveillance Studies.

Section 11. PMA Supplements

Unless noted otherwise below, all procedures and actions that apply to an original PMA also apply to PMA supplements except that the information required in a supplement is limited to that needed to support the change. A PMA supplement and FDA approval are required for changes affecting the safety or effectiveness of the device unless FDA has allowed the information concerning the change to be submitted in an annual report, as discussed above.

The initial decision on whether a PMA supplement is required falls primarily on the PMA holder. However, if the PMA holder does not obtain FDA approval and markets a modified device for which the FDA subsequently determines that the change required a supplement, the device may be found to be adulterated or misbranded, depending on the nature of the change. Therefore, it is always advisable to check with the appropriate review division or the Program Operations Staff in ODE to get advice on whether a PMA supplement is required.

Samples of some of the kinds of changes that may affect safety or effectiveness requiring a PMA supplement include:

- A new indication for use

- Labeling changes

- Changes in the manufacturing facility

- Packaging changes

- Change in the sterilization method

- Performance or design changes

- Extension of an expiration date

A PMA supplement and FDA approval are not required for any change that does not affect safety or effectiveness. As explained above, FDA may require such a change to be reported in the annual report.

Types of PMA Supplements

There are several types of PMA supplements:

- Normal 180-day supplement

- Panel-track supplement

- Real-time supplement

- Special supplement—changes being effected

- 30-day notice, including a 135-day supplement

- Manufacturing site change supplement

Below are brief summaries of the major types of PMA supplements. More-detailed information about PMA supplements can be obtained from the FDA guidance document "Modifications to Devices Subject to Premarket Approval (PMA)—The PMA Supplement Decision-Making Process" which was issued on December 11, 2008. This guidance contains many examples of the types of supplements and the device changes that would be appropriate for consideration under each type of supplement. The guidance is on the FDA website at:

http://www.fda.gov/MedicalDevices/DeviceRegulationand
Guidance/GuidanceDocuments/ucm089274.htm

Normal 180-Day Supplement

A normal 180-day PMA supplement is required for any significant change in an approved device dealing with components, materials, design, specification, software, color additives, or labeling that affects safety and effectiveness. In-depth review and approval by FDA are required before implementation of the change. These supplements usually, but not always, require only new preclinical data unless the data in the original PMA are insufficient to deal with the modification. Sometimes only limited confirmatory clinical data are required. Just as with an original PMA, the supplement should be discussed with FDA prior to its preparation and submission.

Some normal 180-day supplements may be treated as a panel-track supplement or a real-time supplement as discussed immediately below.

Panel-Track Supplement

The term *panel-track supplement* is defined as a supplement that requests a significant change in design or performance of the device, or a new indication for use of the device, for which substantial clinical data are necessary to provide a reasonable assurance of safety and effectiveness. FDA will determine, after receipt of a supplement, whether it in fact meets this threshold, and if it does, the agency will require the review and recommendation of an advisory panel. It is wise to discuss this issue with FDA when such a supplement is being prepared. The panel review process is discussed above in part 1, section 4, Advisory Committee Review and Outside Expertise.

Real-Time Supplement

The term *real-time supplement* is a description used for a supplement that requests a minor change to the device, such as a minor change to the design of the device, software, sterilization, or labeling, and for which the applicant has requested and the agency has granted a meeting or similar forum to jointly review and determine the status of the supplement. This type of supplement is one that does not require new clinical data or a manufacturing site inspection. It involves accepted test methods in one scientific discipline.

In this process, the supplement is reviewed during a meeting or conference call with the applicant. FDA will fax its decision to the applicant within five working days after the meeting or call.

Special Supplement—Changes Being Effected

If the supplement deals with certain manufacturing and labeling changes that enhance the safety of the device or the use of the device, the change may be placed into effect by the applicant prior to the receipt of a written FDA order approving the PMA supplement. Labeling changes must be based on new information that was not available at the time the original PMA was approved, and the information must provide a scientifically legitimate foundation for modifying the FDA-approved labeling. The manufacturing changes that may be reviewed as a special PMA supplement are generally those that add a step to the quality control or manufacturing processes to enhance safety and that do not impact effectiveness.

Before the changes identified in this type of supplement may be placed into effect, the applicant must receive an acknowledgment from FDA that the application has been received by the agency. Furthermore, the PMA supplement and its mailing cover must be plainly marked "special PMA supplement—changes being effected." It must include a full explanation of the basis for the changes, specifically identify the date that such changes are being effected, and confirm that the changes are made according to the Good Manufacturing Practice regulation.

30-Day Notice and 135-Day Supplements

The 30-day notice may be used for modifications to manufacturing procedures or methods of manufacture that affect the safety and effectiveness of the device. These types of changes might be those that reduce manufacturing or labor cost, reduce manufacturing time, reduce waste, or compensate for a change in suppliers of raw material or components. In this case, the change may be made 30 days after FDA receives the 30-day notice unless FDA informs the PMA holder that the 30-day notice is not adequate and describes the additional information or action required.

Certain changes that do not qualify for a 30-day notice include changes in a manufacturing site or sterilization site, or changes to the design or performance specifications. In this case, if the submission contains adequate data for supplemental review, FDA will notify the applicant that the submission is being converted to a 135-day supplement for review. If the submission does not contain adequate data and information, the applicant must submit a normal 180-day supplement.

Manufacturing Site Change Supplement

This type of supplement would be used for a change in the facility or establishment that manufactures, processes, or packages the device. The 180-day supplement is reviewed by the CDRH Office of Compliance or the Office of In Vitro Diagnostic Device Evaluation and Safety for in vitro diagnostic products. FDA will be issuing separate guidance for this type of supplement that describes the criteria for manufacturing site change supplements and when an inspection would likely occur.

Choosing a PMA Supplement

FDA has provided a schematic of the decision-making steps to help in determining which type of supplement is appropriate for changes to an approved PMA device in the guidance document "Modifications to Devices Subject to Premarket Approval (PMA)—The PMA Supplement Decision-Making Process." The flowchart appears in Figure 1.1, "Recommended steps to decide the regulatory path for a modified PMA device" and can be found on the web page cited above under Types of PMA Supplements.

Section 12. Product Development Protocols

Product development protocols, or PDPs, could be thought of as a variant form of a PMA. The PDP must meet the same substantive requirements as a PMA, but the form of the submission is different. The similarity is particularly true in relation to the extent of data required and the rigor of the FDA review. The PDP, just as a PMA, must establish, through valid scientific data and information, that the device is safe and effective. When the PDP has been declared completed by FDA, it is considered to be an approved PMA.

One major difference between a PDP and a PMA is the initiation of the application process. Before starting the PDP process, the sponsor must present the plan to and obtain the agreement of FDA. The PDP is essentially a contract that describes the agreed-on details of design and development activities, the outputs of these activities, and acceptance criteria for these outputs. This allows a sponsor to come to early agreement with FDA as to what may be done to demonstrate the safety and effectiveness of a new device. It also establishes reporting milestones that convey important information to the FDA as it is generated, where they can be reviewed and responded to in a timely manner. This process of early interaction in the development cycle of a device allows a sponsor to address the concerns of the FDA before expensive and time-consuming resources are expended. Ideal candidates for the PDP process are those devices in which the technology is well established in industry. The PDP process provides the manufacturer with the advantage of predictability once the agreement has been reached with FDA.

Section 13. Humanitarian Device Exemptions

The Humanitarian Device Exemption (HDE) was added to the FDCA by Congress to provide incentive for development of devices intended for use, treatment, or diagnosis in small patient populations where a device manufacturer's research and development costs would exceed market returns. The HDE is like a truncated PMA for a very limited purpose, involving a two-step process to obtain marketing approval.

The first step in the process to obtain marketing approval for a device under an HDE is to have the device designated a Humanitarian Use Device (HUD). The second step is to have it approved for marketing under an HDE. The HUD designation is granted by the FDA Office of Orphan Products Development (OOPD), not CDRH. As with other premarket submissions, an HDE is reviewed and approved by CDRH/ODE.

Humanitarian Use Device Designation

To have a device designated a HUD, the sponsor must demonstrate that the device is intended to benefit patients by treating or diagnosing a disease or condition that affects or is manifested in fewer than 4000 individuals in the United States per year. If the disease or condition occurs in more than 4000 patients per year, the device could be used in a subset of the disease or condition as long as the sponsor shows that the subset is "medically plausible" and not just "readily identifiable."

A medically plausible subset is one in which use of the device is limited to that subset because of some inherent property of the device or the disease. That is, the sponsor must explain why the device couldn't also be used in all patients with that disease or condition.

The HDE Application Approval Process

It should be noted at the outset that HDEs are very specialized, and the FDA does not receive many HDE applications. Since 1996, FDA has averaged about four HDEs per year, compared to approximately 5000 510(k)s, 50 PMAs, and 300 IDEs per year.

The HDE format is similar to the format of a PMA, and there may be amendments and supplements. HDE holders have to submit post-market reports and comply with good manufacturing practice requirements and medical device reporting. It is possible to have multiple HDEs approved for the same indication, but once a PMA is approved or a 510(k) is cleared for the same indication for use, no more HDEs will be allowed.

HDE Application Contents

There is one big difference between an HDE application and a PMA. The HDE is not required to contain the results of scientifically valid clinical investigations demonstrating that the device is effective for its intended purpose.

The application, however, must contain sufficient information for FDA to determine that the device does not pose an unreasonable or significant risk of illness or injury and that the probable benefit to health outweighs the risk of injury or illness from its use, taking into account the probable risks and benefits of currently available devices or alternative forms of treatment.

Additionally, the applicant must demonstrate that no comparable devices are available to treat or diagnose the disease or condition, and that they could not otherwise bring the device to market. "Comparable" does not mean identical to the device that is the subject of the HDE.

In addition to the foregoing, the HDE should contain the following elements:

- The HUD designation from the Office of Orphan Products Development

- Information about the device and alternative treatments, if any, including:

  - A device description

  - Published literature on the device

- Nonclinical testing

- Clinical information including:

- Clinical experience, including test data and literature

- Marketing experience outside the United States (OUS)

- Clinical data on the device's use in the patient population, usually from small, uncontrolled studies

- IRB approval

• Information on the disease, including:

- What is known about the disease

- Published literature on the disease

- Disease effects

- Prognosis

• Benefits versus risks in using the device

• Manufacturing information

• Labeling for the physician and the patient

• Labeling that clearly identifies the device as a HUD device and that effectiveness for the indication has not been demonstrated

• The amount to be charged, including a verifying report by an independent certified public accountant or responsible corporate official if the charge is more than $250

FDA Action on an HDE

The approval threshold that will be applied by FDA in determining the approvability of the device is whether (1) the device exposes patients to unreasonable risk of illness or injury, and (2) the probable benefit outweighs the risks of using the device, taking into account the probable risks and benefits of alternative therapies.

Most of the same procedures applicable to PMAs, as described above, are applicable to an HDE. One major difference is that the FDA review times are shorter for an HDE, primarily because the HDE is a less complex and detailed application.

As stated above, a HUD is intended for a patient population that does not exceed 4000 patients per year. The HDE approval order will contain an annual distribution number (ADN), which is based on the number of individuals affected, the number likely to use the device, and the number of devices reasonably necessary to treat such individuals. During any year, the number of devices distributed may not exceed the specified ADN in the HDE approval order.

Examples of HDE approvals include:

- Pediatric left ventricular assist device (LVAD)

- Pediatric pulmonary valved conduit

- Cardiac transplant rejection breath test

- Deep brain stimulator for treatment of intractable chronic dystonia

- Intracerebral stent for treatment of recurrent intracranial stroke

- Intrabronchial valve for sealing air leaks after lung resection surgery

Using a HUD

A practitioner who wishes to use a HUD in the treatment of a patient must first obtain initial and continuing IRB approval in compliance with the IRB regulations.

Use of a HUD for individual patients within approved labeling does not constitute research. However, if data are being collected on another indication, such action would constitute research and require an IDE. No IDE is required for research to collect safety and effectiveness data to support a PMA or a 510(k) if done in accordance with approved labeling. Nevertheless, IRB approval and informed consent are required.

Records

The holders of an approved HDE must maintain (1) records of the names and addresses of the facilities to which a HUD is shipped, (2) correspondence with reviewing IRBs, and (3) any other information required by a reviewing IRB or the FDA.

Profit Making

The amount charged for a HUD can not exceed the cost of research, development, manufacturing, and distribution. The FDCA will allow for a profit to be made only for devices "specifically designed to meet a pediatric need," which provides incentives to manufacturers to develop products specifically designed for use in children. This approach was adopted by Congress because few devices are designed for children's small and growing bodies. Development of children's devices lags five to 10 years behind that of adults, largely due to the limited size of the market for pediatric devices.

HDE Guidance

On July 8, 2010, FDA issued a guidance document entitled "Guidance for HDE Holders, Institutional Review Boards (IRBs), Clinical Investigators, and FDA Staff—Humanitarian Device Exemption (HDE) Regulation: Questions and Answers." This guidance provides detailed information about the HDE program by answering 66 frequently asked questions. The guidance can be accessed at:

> http://www.fda.gov/MedicalDevices/DeviceRegulationand
> Guidance/GuidanceDocuments/ucm110194.htm

PART 4. IMPORTING AND EXPORTING MEDICAL DEVICES FOR COMMERCIAL DISTRIBUTION

Medical devices may be imported or exported for the purpose of commercial distribution or the conduct of a clinical trial. The importation or exportation of an investigational device is covered in Chapter 4, part 7, Importing and Exporting Medical Devices for Investigational Use.

This part deals with the importation or exportation of medical devices for commercial distribution, which is primarily a business marketing decision. Thus, this part provides only an overview of these requirements. Anyone interested in more particulars about importing or exporting a medical device can find detailed information on the following FDA web page. (The quoted materials below come from links on this page.):

> http://www.fda.gov/MedicalDevices/DeviceRegulationand
> Guidance/ImportingandExportingDevices/default.htm

Section 1. Importing a Medical Device

General Rule

FDA can refuse to admit a device into the United States if the device appears to be adulterated or misbranded or if the device is restricted from sale in the country in which it was produced or in the country from which it was exported. In other words, any device imported for domestic distribution must meet all standards applicable to devices produced in the United States. For devices that do not meet U.S. standards, FDA may first give the owner or recipient of the device a chance to recondition the device in order to bring it into compliance with the FDCA.

Foreign Manufacturers

The requirements that apply to foreign manufacturers are stated by FDA in the following manner:

> Foreign manufacturers must meet applicable United States (U.S.) medical device regulations in order to import devices into the U.S. even if the product is authorized for marketing in another country. These requirements include registration of establishment, listing of devices, manufacturing in accordance with the quality system regulation, medical device reporting of adverse events, and Premarket Notification 510(k) or Premarket Approval, if applicable. In addition, the foreign manufacturers must designate a United States agent. As with domestic manufacturers, foreign manufacturing sites are subject to FDA inspection.

Importing Device Components for Subsequent Export

A company can import a component or accessory of a device that is ready or suitable for use for health-related purposes if (1) the importer submits a statement to FDA at the time of initial importation reporting that the imported article is intended to be incorporated into a device that will be lawfully exported, (2) the initial owner or recipient of the component keeps records and, if requested, makes a report to FDA regarding the use or disposition of the imported article, and (3) the owner or consignee destroys or exports any component or accessory that is not incorporated.

The making of a knowingly false statement in any of these required records or reports, the failure to maintain or submit any of the required records or reports, the release into interstate commerce of any of these imported articles or any finished product made from those articles, and the failure to destroy or export any component part or accessory that is not incorporated are prohibited acts.

Section 2. Exporting a Medical Device

Legally Marketed Devices

Devices that comply with all applicable requirements of the FDCA, including registration and listing, marketing approval, labeling, manufacturing requirements, and other general controls, can be exported, just as they may be shipped in domestic commerce, without prior FDA notification or approval. However, there are times when an exporter needs an export certificate from FDA as a requirement by the foreign country to which the device is being exported. FDA explains its policy on issuance of such certificates as follows:

> While FDA does not place any restrictions on the export of these devices, certain countries may require written certification that a firm or its devices are in compliance with U.S. law. In such instances FDA will accommodate U.S. firms by providing a Certificate for Foreign Government (CFG). These export certifications were formerly referred to as a Certificate for Products for Export or Certificate of Free Sale. The CFG is a self-certification process that is used to speed the processing of requests. Original certificates will be provided on special counterfeit-resistant paper with an embossed gold foil seal.

Unapproved Devices

Exporting a medical device that has not been approved or cleared for domestic distribution is governed by a complex set of provisions within Sections 801 and 802 of the FDCA. The following categories of devices for export have their own specific requirements:

1. *An adulterated or misbranded device.* This is a device that does not meet the requirements for domestic marketing. In such a case the device:

   > . . . may be exported legally and without FDA permission in accord with Section 801(e)(1) provided the device is:
   >
   > - in accordance with the specifications of the foreign purchaser;
   > - not in conflict with the laws of the country to which it is intended for export;
   > - labeled on the outside of the shipping package that it is intended for export; and
   > - not sold or offered for sale in domestic commerce.

2. *A non-cleared device.* This is a device that does not have 510(k) clearance, possibly because it will be used strictly for export, or a 510(k) is pending clearance. FDA advises that:

FDA allows the export of a device that does not have a 510(k) marketing clearance without prior FDA clearance if it meets two conditions:

- the device meets the requirements of 801(e)(1) listed above, and

- it is reasonably believed that the device could obtain 510(k) marketing clearance in the U.S. if reviewed by FDA.

3. *A Class III device, performance standard device, or a banned device.* This is a device that lacks a necessary PMA or does not comply with an applicable performance standard, or a banned device. This type of device can be exported with FDA approval, or it can be exported without FDA approval if it meets the conditions in item 1 above. The device must:

- substantially meet Quality Systems *[sic]* Regulation (also known as Good Manufacturing Practices) or an international quality standard recognized by FDA (currently, none are recognized),

- not be adulterated other than by the lack of marketing approval,

- not be the subject of a notice by Department of Health and Human Services that reimportation would pose an imminent hazard, nor pose an imminent hazard to the receiving country, and

- not be mislabeled other than by possessing the language, units of measure, or any other labeling authorized by the recipient country. In addition, the labeling must comply with the requirements and conditions of use in the listed country which gave marketing authorization, and must be promoted in accordance with its labeling.

There are many other specific requirements for exporting a medical device that are described on the FDA page cited above.

FDA Notification

Persons exporting a device under section 802 of the act must provide written notification to FDA. The notification must identify:

- The product's trade name;

- The type of device;

- The product's model number; and

- The country that is to receive the exported article if the export is to a country not listed (non tier 1 country). The notification may, but is not required to, identify the listed (tier 1) countries or may state that the export is intended for a listed (tier 1) country without identifying the listed country.

Because fulfilling the export requirements exempts the device from adulteration and misbranding, a failure to fulfill any of the export requirements renders the device adulterated and/or misbranded.

Device exporters must also maintain certain records, register their facility, and list their devices.

FDA Export Flowchart

The rules for exportation of a medical device are complex. An FDA flowchart to explain the process for determining whether a medical device may be exported can be found at:

http://www.fda.gov/MedicalDevices/DeviceRegulationand
Guidance/ImportingandExportingDevices/ucm050521.
htm#flowchart

PART 5. EXERCISES

1. What are the four major types of premarket submissions that are required prior to the commercial distribution of a medical device in the United States?

2. What constitutes valid scientific evidence that may be used in a 510(k) or PMA? Provide examples of evidence that are acceptable as valid scientific evidence and those that are not acceptable.

3. What is the meaning of the concept "reasonable assurances of safety"?

4. What is the meaning of the concept "reasonable assurances of effectiveness"?

5. What does "substantial equivalence" mean?

6. List the labeling requirements for a medical device.

7. How will the principles of human factors engineering be applied to labeling for a medical device?

8. Name some of the kinds of problems with the data in an application that have resulted in a data integrity action by FDA.

9. What is the purpose of the 510(k) program?

10. Explain the differences between a traditional, special, and abbreviated 510(k).

11. As the director of regulatory affairs, you are informed that the design plan and preclinical testing have been completed for a new daily wear contact lens. You are requested to draft a 510(k) summary for the lens to be submitted to FDA. After checking FDA's 510(k) database for similar devices, the FDA screening checklist, the FDA decision-making flowchart, and the web for sample 510(k)s, please prepare a draft 510(k) summary and presentation for review and approval by the product development committee prior to submission to FDA.

12. What is the purpose and content of a PMA summary?

13 Identify the regulatory compliance statements that must be included in a PMA submission.

14. Explain the purpose and content of the PMA summary of safety and effectiveness data. Examine the FDA database of SSEDs and include the link to the SSED that you think is a good representation of the purpose and intent of this requirement, and explain why.

15. Enumerate the types of changes in an approved PMA device that would necessitate the submission and approval of a PMA supplement, and list the types of PMA supplements.

16. How is a product development protocol similar to and different from a PMA?

17. What are the conditions that must be met for a device to be designated a humanitarian use device (HUD) that is eligible for approval under a humanitarian device exemption?

6

Post-Market Requirements

One of the purposes of premarket review is to evaluate information on a device's safety and effectiveness to determine whether the device may be introduced into interstate commerce for commercial distribution. However, there may be questions that can not be answered during the premarket review process, or an issue may arise after the device is marketed. The need for enhanced post-market vigilance is driven by the pervasive use of medical devices and their potential to do harm as well as good. For example: devices are becoming more complex and smaller, which leaves less margin for error; implanted devices are being used for longer periods of time and in younger populations; and post-market safety assessment is hampered by insufficient numerator and denominator information because of severe underreporting and limited or lacking denominator information. See discussion of device failures in Chapter 2, part 7, Design Failures.

Accordingly, the Food, Drug, and Cosmetic Act (FDCA) provides a number of tools to protect the public health while continuing the availability of safe and effective medical devices. Under the act and its implementing regulations, a manufacturer has a responsibility to monitor the post-market use of its products to assure the continued safe use of the products. Since December 13, 1984, the FDA Medical Device Reporting (MDR) regulations have required firms who have received complaints of device malfunctions, serious injuries, or deaths associated with medical devices to notify FDA of the incident. The Safe Medical Devices Act (SMDA) of 1990 provided FDA and industry with two additional post-marketing tools: *post-market surveillance* for the monitoring of products in the marketplace, and *device tracking* for maintaining traceability of certain devices to the user level. Lastly, the agency may order a manufacturer to notify users of problems with its device or to render repair, replacement, or refund. This chapter discusses each of these topics.

When a manufacturer discovers a problem with a marketed device, it must correct the problem or remove the device from the distribution chain. If the defect that requires correction or removal renders the device a violative product, the action is referred to as a *recall*. Recalls may be voluntarily initiated by the manufacturer as provided in the FDCA, or they may be mandated by FDA. Both of these recalls are discussed in this chapter. The mandatory recall would be appropriate for discussion in Chapter 8, Compliance and Enforcement, but it is included here with voluntary recalls rather than discussing recalls in two different places. This avoids duplication and facilitates an integrated discussion.

Other post-market responsibilities that manufacturers have are discussed in other chapters of the book because they derive from, or fit naturally within, the topics discussed there. For example, the responsibility of a manufacturer to notify FDA of certain labeling changes made after the device is approved for marketing is discussed in Chapter 5, part 2, Premarket Notification (510[k]) and part 3, PMAs/PDPs/HDEs. Likewise, submitting annual reports and conducting post-approval studies is discussed in Chapter 5, part 3, PMAs/PDPs/HDEs.

PART 1. MEDICAL DEVICE REPORTING

The Medical Device Reporting regulation provides a mechanism for FDA to identify and monitor significant adverse events involving marketed medical devices. The goal of the MDR program is to detect and correct after-market problems in a timely manner. It provides a mechanism for the FDA to obtain significant medical device adverse events from manufacturers, importers, and user facilities. For this program to be effective, it requires the goodwill and cooperation of all affected groups to accomplish the objectives of the program.

Section 1. Applicability and Reportable Events

The MDR regulation requires manufacturers, importers, and user facilities to report, using FDA MedWatch forms, significant medical device adverse events from marketed medical devices. Each of these reporters has slightly different responsibilities, which are discussed below. There are three basic types of events that have to be reported:

- Deaths
- Serious injury or illness

- Device malfunction or failure

Serious Injury/Serious Illness

A serious injury or serious illness is one that:

- Is life-threatening, even if temporary in nature

- Results in permanent impairment of a body function or permanent damage to a body structure, or

- Necessitates medical or surgical intervention to preclude permanent impairment of a body function or permanent damage to a body structure

Device Malfunction

A malfunction is a failure of the device to meet its performance specifications or otherwise perform as intended. Performance specifications include all claims made in the labeling for the device. The essential function of a device includes not only the device's labeled use, but any use widely prescribed within the practice of medicine. A malfunction should be considered reportable if any one of the following is true:

- The chance of a death or serious injury occurring as a result of a recurrence of the malfunction is not remote.

- The consequences of the malfunction affect the device in a catastrophic manner that may lead to a death or serious injury.

- It causes the device to fail to perform its essential function and compromises the device's therapeutic, monitoring, or diagnostic effectiveness, which could cause or contribute to a death or serious injury, or causes other significant adverse device experiences.

- It involves the malfunction of an implant that would be likely to cause or contribute to death or serious injury, regardless of how the device is used.

- The device is considered life-supporting or life-sustaining, and thus essential to maintaining human life.

- The manufacturer would be required, as a result of the malfunction of the device or other similar devices, to issue a notification of the malfunction, repair or replace the device, make a refund or reimbursement to the purchaser, make a correction to the device, or remove it from distribution, including initiating a recall, except for routine servicing.

Reporters do not need to assess the likelihood that a malfunction will occur again. The regulation presumes that the malfunction will recur. Furthermore, FDA believes that once a malfunction has caused or contributed to a death or serious injury, a presumption that the malfunction is likely to cause or contribute to a death or serious injury has been established. This presumption will continue until the malfunction has caused or contributed to no further deaths or serious injuries for two years, or the manufacturer can show, through valid data, that the likelihood of another death or serious injury as a result of the malfunction is remote.

Not all malfunctions are reportable. Malfunctions are not reportable if they are not likely to result in a death, serious injury, or other significant adverse event experience. Also, a malfunction that is or can be corrected during routine service or device maintenance must be reported only if the recurrence of the malfunction is likely to cause or contribute to a death or serious injury.

Section 2. Reporting Responsibilities

The MDR regulation requires manufacturers, importers, and user facilities to report significant medical device adverse events from marketed medical devices. Each of the persons required to report deaths, serious injury or illness, or device malfunctions has slightly different responsibilities as discussed in this section.

User Facilities

The term *user facility* includes a hospital, an ambulatory surgical facility, a nursing home, a skilled nursing facility, a hospice care center, a rehabilitation center, an outpatient diagnostic facility, or any other outpatient treatment facility, unless specifically exempted by the regulation. A physician's office, school nurse offices, and employee health units are not device user facilities under this regulation.

- *Deaths.* User facilities are required to report device-related deaths to the FDA and the manufacturer within 10 working days of a death.

- *Serious injury or illness.* They must submit reports of serious injuries only to the manufacturer. However, if the manufacturer is unknown, reports of serious injuries must be submitted to FDA.

- *Device malfunctions or failures.* The user facility is not required, but is encouraged, to report reportable malfunctions to the manufacturer.

- In addition, user facilities must submit to FDA on an annual basis a summary of all reports submitted during that period.

These reporting requirements for user facilities are summarized in Table 6.1.

Distributors

Distributors are persons who sell medical devices to other sellers or users but do not manufacture the devices or repackage or otherwise change the container, wrapper, or labeling of the device or device package. Under the MDR regulation, a distributor must maintain records of incidents, but it is not required to report these incidents. It must establish and maintain device complaint records or files. These records must contain any incident information, including any written, electronic, or oral communication, either received or generated by the distributor, that alleges deficiencies related to the identity (for example, labeling), quality, durability, reliability, safety, effectiveness, or performance of a device. A distributor must also maintain information about the evaluation of the allegations, if any, in the incident record. The records may be in written or electronic format and must be identified as device incident records and filed by device name.

Importers

An importer of medical devices must report each individual adverse event as soon as practicable but no later than 30 calendar days after the day that the reportable event becomes known. The importer must submit a MedWatch Form 3500A report of each device-related death or serious injury to FDA

Table 6.1 Summary of reporting requirements for user facilities.

Reporter	What to report	MedWatch report form #	To whom	When
User facility	Death	Form FDA 3500A	FDA and manufacturer	Within 10 work days
User facility	Serious injury	Form FDA 3500A	Manufacturer—FDA only if manufacturer unknown	Within 10 work days
User facility	Annual reports of death and serious injury	Form FDA 3419	FDA	January 1

and to the manufacturer. Reports of device-related malfunctions must be submitted to the manufacturer.

Manufacturers and U.S. Agents of Foreign Manufacturers

Under the MDR regulation, all manufacturers, which include by definition the U.S. agents of foreign manufacturers, must report to FDA whenever a device:

- May have caused or contributed to a death or serious injury, or

- Has malfunctioned and would be likely to cause or contribute to a death or serious injury if the malfunction were to recur

The type of event must be reported to FDA within 30 days of the time the manufacturer becomes aware of the event. If a reportable event requires remedial action to prevent an unreasonable risk of substantial harm to the public health, it must be reported within five days. These reporting requirements for manufacturers are summarized in Table 6.2.

It is safe to say that most, if not all, manufacturers receive complaints about their products from time to time. In the case of medical devices, each manufacturer must review and evaluate all complaints to determine whether any complaint represents an event that must be reported to FDA.

For manufacturers that market a PMA-approved device, it is important to note that the same events subject to reporting under the MDR regulation may also be subject to the "adverse reaction and device defect reporting" requirements if the "conditions of approval" for the PMA contain such a requirement. FDA does not want to receive duplicative reports. Whenever an event occurs involving a device that is subject to reporting under both the MDR regulation and the "Adverse Reaction Report" or "Device Defect Report" in the conditions of approval for the PMA, the applicant must submit the report on the MedWatch form as required by the MDR regulation. In doing so, the manufacturer would include the PMA reference number on the MedWatch form. To comply with the PMA condition, the manufacturer need only include in its annual report under the PMA an identification of the MDR-reported events. This process of referencing prevents duplicative entries into FDA's information systems. Adverse reaction and device defect reporting are discussed in Chapter 5, part 3, PMAs/PDPs/HDEs. As stated there, FDA is no longer including the adverse reaction and device defect reporting requirement in PMA approval letters, so the problem of duplicate reporting will eventually disappear.

An extensive FDA guidance, "Medical Device Reporting for Manufacturers," can be found at:

Table 6.2 Summary of reporting requirements for manufacturers.

Reporter	What to report	Report form #	To whom	When
Manufacturer	30-day reports of deaths, serious injuries, and malfunctions.	Form FDA 3500A	FDA	Within 30 calendar days of becoming aware of an event.
Manufacturer	Five-day reports on events that require remedial action to prevent an unreasonable risk of substantial harm to the public health, and other types of events designated by FDA.	Form FDA 3500A	FDA	Within five workdays of becoming aware of an event.
Manufacturer	Baseline reports to identify and provide basic data on each device that is the subject of an MDR report. At this time, FDA has stayed the requirement for denominator data requested in Part II, items 15 and 16, on Form 3417.	Form FDA 3417	FDA	With 30-calendar, and five-workday reports when device or device family is reported for the first time. Interim and annual updates are also required if any baseline information changes after initial submission.
Manufacturer	Annual certification.	Form FDA 3381	FDA	Coincides with firm's annual registration dates.

http://www.fda.gov/MedicalDevices/DeviceRegulationand
Guidance/GuidanceDocuments/ucm094529.htm#elect

FDA Forms

FDA has two forms for reporting MDRs, one for voluntary reporting and one for mandatory reporting. Healthcare professionals, consumers, and patients may voluntarily report adverse events on FDA Form 3500. All parties that must report to FDA under MDR must use FDA Form 3500A. Copies of these forms along with instructions can be obtained from the FDA website at:

http://www.fda.gov/Safety/MedWatch/HowToReport/
DownloadForms/default.htm

These forms can be filled out on a computer using the Adobe Acrobat Reader. They also may be printed and filled out by hand. The voluntary Form FDA 3500 features a postage-paid pre-addressed mailer.

Form 3500A is required for each device involved in a mandatory reportable event. For example, if a manufacturer receives a report from a user facility that indicates that more than one of the manufacturer's devices may have been involved in a reportable event, a separate report from the manufacturer to FDA for each device is required. A report is required when a manufacturer becomes aware of information that reasonably suggests that one of its marketed devices has or may have caused or contributed to a death or serious injury, or has malfunctioned, and that the device or a similar device marketed by the manufacturer would be likely to cause or contribute to a death or serious injury if the malfunction were to recur. In cases where the manufacturer receives information regarding a reportable event other than by means of a Form 3500A, they are required to complete all applicable sections of the form.

Electronic Medical Device Reporting

FDA encourages the use of electronic filings for MDR reports. The agency has provided the following guidance on "eMDR" reports in the guidance cited above:

> Manufacturers may send MDR reports electronically once they have received written approval from FDA. This includes the use of electronic media such as magnetic tape, disc, and computer-to-computer communication. FDA encourages manufacturers to computerize the required report forms. However, a request for an electronic facsimile (reproduction) approval of any form must be made in writing to FDA. The request must include a copy of the proposed form and a sample of a completed form. It is not necessary for a facsimile form to be generated as a two-sided document. Manufacturers can use programs that automatically create continuation pages when the text exceeds the space allowed for a particular block on a form. FDA is not accepting facsimiles that increase the size of the item block or cause the original form to be

significantly modified. The request for facsimile approval should be addressed to the MedWatch address designated below. A copy of all the requests for Form 3500 or Form 3500A approval should be forwarded to the Director, Division of Surveillance Systems at the address designated below.

Section 3. Standard Operating Procedures for MDR

Manufacturers are required to establish and maintain written procedures for implementation of the MDR regulation. These procedures should include internal systems that:

- Provide for timely and effective identification, communication, and evaluation of adverse events

- Provide a standardized review process and procedures for determining whether or not an event is reportable

- Provide procedures to ensure the timely transmission of complete reports

These procedures should also include documentation and record-keeping requirements for:

- Information that was evaluated to determine if an event was reportable

- All medical device reports and information submitted to FDA

- Any information that was evaluated during preparation of annual certification reports

- Systems that ensure access to information that facilitates timely follow-up and inspection by FDA

Each manufacturer has certain discretion to decide the detail and depth of information that its written MDR procedures contain. FDA suggests that manufacturers provide policy and procedure information regarding "typical" adverse events or product problems that may be MDR reportable.

The procedures should describe the investigation protocol that will be followed, for example, the number of attempts that will be made to contact the reporter either by phone, fax, or letter before the investigation is closed, that the complaint records will contain a concise yet thorough description of the adverse event or product problem, that the complaint records will be legible, and so on.

The number of follow-ups necessary to obtain MDR information depends on the nature and severity of the event reported. MDR follow-up investigations should focus on obtaining information and not on the number of attempts. FDA does not provide an absolute number of attempts to follow up since the intensity, nature, and duration of an MDR follow-up depends on the firm's assessment of the risk. Therefore, "adequate" follow-up can not be characterized by the selection of a predetermined/averaged number of attempts. Each MDR event can be unique, and a standard number of follow-up attempts would not be in the best interest of the public health.

Each manufacturer must make a "good faith effort" to obtain information. At least one request for information should be made in writing. Firms must document follow-up attempts and document reasons why MDR information can not be obtained. A firm's files should include a record of each attempt to obtain information and the nature of the response by the reporter. All of this information will be reviewed by FDA to determine if a firm has made a reasonable attempt to follow up and obtain the required information.

Section 4. Record-Keeping Requirements

Manufacturers must maintain complete MDR files in either written or electronic form. They must identify them prominently as "MDR files" so they can be found easily. Manufacturers' MDR files may be maintained as part of their complaint files required under the Quality System Regulation (QSR). An MDR report submitted to FDA is not considered in compliance with the MDR regulation unless the manufacturer evaluated the event in accordance with the QSR regarding investigation of a possible device failure. There must be a record of this investigation documented in the complaint file. See Chapter 7, part 11, Records, for a discussion of the QSR records and complaint files required under QSR.

Content of MDR Records

MDR files must contain information related to the event, including all documentation of deliberations and decision-making processes used to decide whether the event was or was not reportable, and the original or a copy of the initial complaint/event record. This record should include the available information needed to complete the Form 3500A. The record may be a documented telephone call, a letter or fax, a service report, documents related to a lawsuit, a voluntary Form 3500 received from a healthcare professional or consumer, or a mandatory Form 3500A received from a user facility or a distributor. The records should also include:

- Copies of any records documenting the firm's attempts to follow up and obtain missing or additional information about the event, including an explanation of why any missing information was not obtained and submitted

- Copies of any test reports, laboratory reports, service records and reports, and records of investigations

- Copies of all documentation involving the final assessment of the event, any deliberation or decision-making processes used to determine whether an MDR report was or was not needed, and what action the firm took to assure that the cause of the event is corrected or otherwise mitigated

- Copies of all 3500As submitted to FDA, when applicable, including a copy of any 3500As received from user facilities and distributors

- Documents verifying that the event has been evaluated in accordance with the applicable requirements of QSR, and

- References to any other relevant documents or information used during the assessment

Record Retention Period

Manufacturers are to maintain records related to an event, whether reportable or not, for two years from the date of the event or a period equivalent to the expected life of the device, whichever is longer. MDR files may incorporate references to other information sources such as medical records, patient files, and engineering reports.

FDA Inspections

Manufacturers must permit any authorized FDA employee to access, copy, and verify the records in the MDR files.

Section 5. Exemptions, Variances, and Alternative Reporting Requirements

The Medical Device Regulation includes provisions for waivers from all or some of its provisions. The regulation explicitly exempts the following three types of persons:

- Licensed practitioners who prescribe or administer devices intended for use in humans, and who manufacture or import devices solely for use in diagnosing and treating persons with whom the practitioner has a "physician–patient" relationship

- A person who manufactures devices intended for use in humans solely for such person's use in research or teaching and not for sale, including any person who is subject to alternative reporting requirements under the investigational device exemption (IDE) regulation because they are conducting a clinical research study

- Dental or optical laboratories

In addition, manufacturers can submit requests for exemption from all or part of the requirements of the MDR. This includes variances and alternative reporting requirements. FDA must approve a manufacturer's request in writing before an exemption, variance, or alternative reporting can be carried out. An exemption, variance, or alternative report approval may also be granted at the discretion of FDA in the absence of a request. FDA can revoke any approval in writing if it decides that the protection of the public health justifies a return to the standard MDR reporting requirements.

A variance may include a modification of the data elements required on the mandatory reporting forms. An alternative report allows a modification in the timing of report submissions and is a type of variance. For example, a firm may request—instead of reporting each event within 30 days after becoming aware of it—that the reports be submitted every two months, quarterly, semiannually, or annually.

When an exemption, variance, or alternative report is granted, FDA may impose other reporting requirements to protect the public health. Manufacturers must provide any reports or information required by FDA in approving any reporting modifications. The conditions of approval replace or supersede the reporting requirements of the MDR.

Section 6. Public Disclosure of MDR Information

FDA maintains a searchable database of all reports on devices that may have malfunctioned or caused a death or serious injury. The files contain both reports received under the MDR program from 1984 to 1996 and the voluntary reports up to June 1993. The database currently contains over 600,000 reports. This information can be accessed and searched through the following FDA website as well as other sources that are referenced at:

http://www.fda.gov/MedicalDevices/Safety/ReportaProblem/ucm124073.htm

Before entering data into the public database, FDA deletes nondisclosable information such as trade secret and confidential commercial information, personal, medical, and similar information, and certain other information about persons making reports under MDR.

PART 2. POST-MARKET SURVEILLANCE STUDIES

In Chapter 5, part 3, PMAs/PDPs/HDEs, post-approval studies are discussed. Those are studies that are required by FDA in a PMA approval order. However, there are times when FDA becomes aware of issues with a device that is already on the market for which further study is indicated. When this occurs, FDA is authorized by the FDCA to order the conduct of a post-market surveillance study of any Class II or Class III device as specified in the act. Pursuant to this authority, FDA promulgated a regulation on post-market surveillance. This part deals with these regulatory post-market surveillance studies.

Post-market surveillance (PS) means the active, systematic, scientifically valid collection, analysis, and interpretation of data or other information about a marketed device. The Postmarket Surveillance Studies Program encompasses design, tracking, oversight, and review responsibilities for studies mandated under this regulation. The program helps ensure that well-designed post-market surveillance studies are conducted effectively and efficiently and in the least burdensome manner.

The Postmarket Surveillance Studies Program for medical devices is managed by the CDRH Office of Surveillance and Biometrics (OSB). Additional information on this program and its requirements can be found in the guidance document "Postmarket Surveillance under Section 522 of the Federal Food, Drug and Cosmetic Act" at the following link:

http://www.fda.gov/MedicalDevices/DeviceRegulationand
Guidance/GuidanceDocuments/ucm072517.htm

Section 1. Applicability and Scope

The Requirement to Conduct Post-Market Surveillance

FDA may require a manufacturer to conduct post-market surveillance of a Class II or Class III device that meets any of the following criteria:

- Failure of the device would be reasonably likely to have serious adverse health consequences.

- The device is intended to be implanted in the human body for more than one year.

- The device is intended to be used outside a user facility to support or sustain life.

Failure to comply with requirements of a PS order will result in the device being considered misbranded.

When a PS study is required, FDA will issue an order in the form of a letter to the manufacturer requiring post-market surveillance. Manufacturers must submit a PS plan for approval within 30 days of receiving an order to conduct a post-market surveillance study from FDA. After receiving the manufacturer's proposed plan, FDA has 60 days to determine if the person designated to conduct the surveillance is qualified and experienced, and whether the plan will collect useful data that can reveal unforeseen adverse events or other information necessary to protect the public health.

Conditions Underlying a PS Order

Post-market issues may be identified through a variety of sources, including analysis of adverse event reports, a recall or corrective action, reports from other governmental authorities, or the scientific literature.

FDA's guidance document "Postmarket Surveillance under Section 522 of the Federal Food, Drug and Cosmetic Act," as cited above, lists the following examples of situations that may raise post-market questions, during both the premarket and post-market periods:

> • *New or expanded conditions of use for existing devices.* [FDA] may order postmarket surveillance to augment premarket data to obtain more experience with change from hospital use to use in the home or other environment or with new patient populations.
> • *Significant changes in device characteristics (technology).* [FDA] may have questions that arise from significant or developmental changes to device technology that can be most appropriately addressed in the postmarket period. The agency may also have concerns that changes in the technology of a device may affect the duration of the effectiveness of the device, which could be addressed by postmarket surveillance. In these situations, postmarket surveillance, through collection of longer-term safety and effectiveness data, may augment premarket data and allow earlier marketing of new technologies without compromising the public health.
> • *Longer-term follow-up or evaluation of rare events.* [The agency] may order postmarket surveillance to address longer-term or less common safety and effectiveness issues of implantable and other devices for which the premarket testing provided only limited information. For example, premarket evaluation of the device may have been based on surrogate markers. Once the device is

actually marketed, postmarket surveillance may be appropriate to assess the effectiveness of the device in detecting or treating the disease or condition, rather than the surrogate. Data collected during postmarket surveillance may include rates of malfunction or failure of a device intended for long-term use or incidents of latent sequelae resulting from device use.

• *Public health concern(s) resulting from reported or suspected problems in marketed devices.* [FDA] may order postmarket surveillance to better define the association between problems and devices when unexpected or unexplained serious adverse events occur after a device is marketed; if there is a change in the nature of serious adverse events (e.g., severity); or if there is an increase in the frequency of serious adverse events.

Factors Affecting the Issuance of a PS Order

FDA may also consider the following factors when determining whether to issue a PS order:

- The ability of other post-market mechanisms to address public health concerns raised by the post-market question, such as PMA post-approval requirements, medical device reports, quality systems requirements, field inspections, or special controls for Class II devices.

- The practicality of post-market surveillance strategies, including the feasibility and timeliness of post-market surveillance. For example, the relative value of post-market surveillance for a given device may be influenced by the rate of device evolution. Post-market surveillance may not be reasonable if the applicability of the results will be minimal by the time post-market surveillance is completed.

- The priority of the post-market question, based on the perceived magnitude of the risk, such as an identified or suspected significant risk to public health.

Section 2. The PS Submission and PS Plan

The Post-Market Surveillance Submission

Upon the receipt of a PS order, the manufacturer must send a post-market surveillance submission to FDA for review and approval. The submission must include the following elements:

- Organizational/administrative information:
  - Manufacturer's name and address
  - Generic and trade names of the device
  - Name and address of the contact person for the submission
  - Premarket application/submission numbers for the device
  - Table of contents identifying the page numbers for each section of the submission
  - Description of the device (this may be incorporated by reference to the appropriate premarket application/submission)
  - Product codes and a list of all relevant model numbers
  - Indications for use and claims for the device
- Post-market surveillance plan
- The following information about the person designated to conduct the surveillance must also be included:
  - Name, address, and telephone number
  - Experience and qualifications

The Surveillance Plan

The surveillance plan contained in the PS submission is not the same as, but is analogous to, the other protocols discussed elsewhere in this book for nonclinical and clinical studies, and must include a discussion of:

- The plan objective(s) addressing the surveillance question(s) identified in the order
- The subject of the study, for example, patients, the device, animals
- The variables and end points that will be used to answer the surveillance question, for example, clinical parameters or outcomes
- The surveillance approach or methodology to be used
- Sample size and units of observation
- The investigator agreement, if applicable
- Sources of data, for example, hospital records
- The data collection plan and forms

- The consent document, if applicable

- Institutional review board information, if applicable

- The patient follow-up plan, if applicable

- The procedures for monitoring conduct and progress of the surveillance

- An estimate of the duration of surveillance

- All data analyses and statistical tests planned

- The content and timing of reports

Methods of Surveillance

Manufacturers may use the most practical and least burdensome approach to produce a scientifically sound answer to the question to be addressed by the post-market surveillance study. FDA provides the following examples to illustrate a range of surveillance methods, and situations in which they might be appropriate:

- *Detailed review of complaint history and scientific literature.* Example: compilation and comparison of the manufacturer's complaint files and published literature to verify frequency of reported adverse events.

- *Nonclinical testing of the device.* Example: analysis of devices explanted from animal models to assess long-term effects of the body on implant materials.

- *Telephone or mail follow-up of a defined patient sample.* Example: evaluation of the effectiveness of user training for a home-use device previously used only in the hospital setting; outcomes easily and reliably reportable directly by patient.

- *Use of secondary data sets (e.g., Medicare), registries (e.g., Society for Interventional Radiology stent registry), internal registries, or tracking systems.* Example: analysis of patient outcomes or device usage. (In these instances, it is important to ensure that variables of interest are included in the data set/registry).

- *Case-control study of patients implanted with or using devices.* Example: comparison of cases and controls to quantify magnitude of risk posed by device exposure.

- *Consecutive enrollment studies.* Example: assessment of outcomes following device exposure, to assess the frequency of problems based on clinical follow-up of patients.

- *Cross-sectional studies (multiple cohorts).* Example: assessment of device safety and/or effectiveness at designated time intervals after the initiation of the postmarket surveillance plan.
  - *Non-randomized controlled cohort studies.* Example: analysis of risks and benefits associated with each of several devices used to treat same disease or condition.
  - *Randomized controlled trials.* Example: evaluate the risk/benefit relationship for a sub-population using a device that has been approved for use with a broad indication.

Section 3. FDA Actions

FDA Review Team

During the process of determining whether to order a PS study, FDA will identify a review team for the surveillance plan. The team will consist of a review team leader from OSB and two or more consulting reviewers from other program offices in CDRH. Each team will consist of, at a minimum, a statistician and/or an epidemiologist, and an ODE premarket reviewer. FDA will add consulting reviewers with expertise relevant to the PS question, for example, human factors, drug elution, or engineering, as appropriate. These reviewers will typically be from the other program offices in CDRH. On occasion, the agency may use staff from other Centers or special government employees (SGEs) if they possess expertise necessary and relevant to the surveillance.

Review Actions

FDA has 60 days to review and respond to PS submissions. In doing so, FDA may issue various interim communications such as deficiency letters or requests for additional information, just as it does during the review of other types of submissions to the agency.

FDA considers the PS complete when the manufacturer has answered the PS questions specified in the surveillance order. If the results of the surveillance raise new issues or questions, additional actions may be required. For example, FDA may:

- Request changes to the labeling of the device to reflect additional information learned from the post-market surveillance

- Issue a new PS order to address a new issue, or

- Consider administrative or regulatory actions if necessary to protect the public health

Release of Information

Under the Freedom of Information Act, most of the information in the PS plan is subject to public release. FDA posts the overall status of the surveillance, along with a brief description of the plan, on the Internet. A listing of Section 522 PS studies can be found at the following website:

> http://www.accessdata.fda.gov/scripts/cdrh/cfdocs/cfPMA/pss.cfm

As with all other submissions to FDA, trade secret and confidential commercial information, as well as any personal identifier information for patients, will be protected from release to the public.

PART 3. MEDICAL DEVICE TRACKING

FDA has the authority under the FDCA to order manufacturers to implement a tracking system for a specific type of device and to track it from its manufacture through the distribution chain. The purpose of device tracking is to ensure that manufacturers of certain devices establish tracking systems that will enable them to promptly locate devices in commercial distribution. Tracking information may be used to facilitate notifications and recalls ordered by FDA in the case of serious risks to health presented by the devices. Tracking augments FDA's authority to order mandatory recalls, as discussed below in part 4, Medical Device Recalls, and require notification of health professionals and patients regarding unreasonable risk of substantial harm associated with a device, which is presented below in part 5, Notification and Three R's.

Section 1. Applicability and Scope

Tracked Devices

The Food and Drug Administration may issue an order to the manufacturer to require the adoption of a method of tracking a Class II or Class III device if the device meets one of the following three criteria:

- The failure of the device would be reasonably likely to have serious adverse health consequences.

- The device is intended to be implanted in the human body for more than one year.

- The device is a life-sustaining or life-supporting device used outside a device user facility.

These criteria are the same as the criteria for requiring a post-approval surveillance study.

The following additional factors may be considered in determining whether a tracking order should be issued:

- The likelihood of a sudden, catastrophic failure

- The likelihood of a significant adverse clinical outcome

- The need for prompt professional intervention

FDA may base its determination on information arising from the review of premarket applications, recall data, medical device reporting, inspections, petitions, post-market surveillance studies, or other information coming to its attention. A device that meets one of these criteria and is the subject of an FDA tracking order is known as a "tracked device."

Responsible Parties

The tracking regulations are intended to ensure that tracked devices can be traced from the device manufacturing facility to the person for whom the device is indicated, that is, the patient. Effective tracking of devices from the manufacturing facility, through the distributor network (including distributors, retailers, rental firms and other commercial enterprises, device user facilities, and licensed practitioners), and, ultimately, to the patient is necessary for the effectiveness of remedies prescribed by the act, such as patient notification or device recall.

Failure of the manufacturer or any distributor in the distribution chain to meet the tracking requirements will cause the device to be misbranded.

In addition to the manufacturer and its distributors, the importer of a tracked device is treated the same as a manufacturer and is required to comply with all of the tracking requirements applicable to manufacturers. Importers must keep all required tracking information in the United States.

The tracking regulations do not preclude a manufacturer from involving outside organizations in that manufacturer's device tracking efforts.

Section 2. Devices Subject to Tracking

Pursuant to its authority under the tracking regulation FDA has issued orders to manufacturers, who are required to track the following lists of implantable devices and devices used outside of a device user facility.

Implantable Devices Requiring Tracking

- Glenoid fossa prosthesis

- Mandibular condyle prosthesis

- Temporomandibular joint (TMJ) prosthesis

- Abdominal aortic aneurysm stent grafts

- Automatic implantable cardioverter/defibrillator

- Cardiovascular permanent implantable pacemaker electrode

- Implantable pacemaker pulse generator

- Replacement heart valve (mechanical only)

- Implanted cerebellar stimulator

- Implanted diaphragmatic/phrenic nerve stimulator

- Implantable infusion pumps

- Dura mater

Devices Used outside of a Device User Facility Requiring Tracking

- Breathing frequency monitors

- Continuous ventilators

- DC defibrillators and paddles

- Ventricular bypass (assist) device

Section 3. The Tracking Process

The purpose of the tracking regulation is to provide certain critical information about the location of a tracked device within a short time frame. No specific method of tracking is required, so manufacturers may have different tracking methods and procedures. All manufacturers, however, must have written standard operating procedures for a method of tracking that will produce the information required by the regulation.

If a manufacturer uses an outside firm to manage its tracking program, the manufacturer is responsible for making sure the outside firm meets the tracking requirements. Manufacturers can not alter, change, or in any way avoid their tracking obligation unless FDA approves a manufacturer's written request for a variance or an exemption.

Manufacturers' Audits

Manufacturers must make sure their method of tracking works. Manufacturers must perform audits at six-month intervals for the first three years a device is tracked, and then annually after three years. Audits should verify that the tracking method actually works and that the information collected is accurate. FDA requires the use of a recognized statistical sampling plan and suggests one such as MIL-STD-105E. Audits may be conducted through on-site visits or through some other effective way of communication with the distributors, professionals, and patients involved.

Section 4. Records and Reports

Distributor Information

For all tracked devices, the manufacturer must maintain the following distributor information:

- Distributors' names

- Distributors' addresses

- Telephone numbers of distributors and the devices' locations

Single-Use Devices

In addition to distributor information, manufacturers are required to obtain and maintain additional information for two types of devices: (1) devices that are life sustaining or life supporting, and used outside a user facility, that are intended for use by a single patient over the life of the device, and (2) devices permanently implanted in a patient for more than one year. The following information must be maintained for each individually tracked device:

- The device's identification (lot, batch, model, or serial number)

- The date the device was shipped by the manufacturer

- The name, address, telephone number, and social security number of the patient who received the device

- The date it was provided to the patient

- The name, mailing address, and telephone number of the prescribing physician

- The name, mailing address, and telephone number of the physician following the patient, if different than the prescribing physician

- The date of the device's explantation, if applicable, and the name, mailing address, and telephone number of the explanting physician, the date of the patient's death, or the date that the device was returned to the manufacturer, permanently retired from use, or otherwise disposed of permanently

Multiple-Use Devices

Manufacturers are not required to obtain and maintain the identity of each patient that uses a tracked device when the device is intended to be used by more than one patient over the useful life of the device. Manufacturers must have a current record relating to the multiple distributor, that is, the one who distributes the device for use by multiple patients, who has the device, and must provide in 10 working days to FDA, upon request, the following information:

- The lot, batch, model, or serial number of the device or other identifier necessary to provide for effective tracking of the device

- The date the device was shipped by the manufacturer

- The name, address, and telephone number of the multiple distributor

- The name, address, telephone number, and social security number, if available, of the patient using the device

- The location of the device

- The date the device was provided to a patient for use

- The name, address, and telephone number of the prescribing physician

- If and when applicable, the date that the device was returned to the manufacturer, permanently retired from use, or otherwise disposed of permanently or remarketed

Reports to FDA

Manufacturers will have three days to provide critical information about devices that have not yet been distributed to a patient, and 10 working days for devices that have been distributed to patients.

PART 4. MEDICAL DEVICE RECALLS

After a medical device is distributed, the manufacturer or distributor of the device may discover a defect or malfunction of the device that requires correcting the problem or removing the product from the distribution chain. Such correction or removal may constitute a recall depending on whether the device was in violation of a regulatory requirement. This part discusses the differences between a market withdrawal and a recall, the classification of recalls, and the differences between a voluntary and mandatory recall. Recall information is important to members of the medical device industry because they can glean information that may be useful in their design efforts (including HFE factors), in their manufacturing processes, or in constructing effective instructions for use.

There are several sources with detailed information on the regulations and actions related to recalls. The FDA "Guidance for Industry: Product Recalls, Including Removals and Corrections," which covers recalls for all types of FDA-regulated products, can be found at:

> http://www.fda.gov/Safety/Recalls/IndustryGuidance/ucm 129259.htm

For lists of device recalls see the following websites:

> http://www.fda.gov/MedicalDevices/Safety/RecallsCorrections Removals/ListofRecalls/default.htm

> http://www.fda.gov/Safety/Recalls/default.htm

Section 1. Corrections and Removals

Device corrections or removals by firms are frequently an early signal to FDA that a post-market device problem may exist. Table 6.3 lists the types of actions that qualify as a correction or a removal. As the table demonstrates, the same actions may qualify as either a correction or removal depending on whether the device is removed from the point of use.

A correction or removal may be due to manufacturing problems, materials quality issues, device design issues, incomplete labeling, or a user

Table 6.3   Making a device correction or removal.

"Correction"—without physical removal of the device from point of use:	"Removal"—physical removal of a device from point of use for:
Repair	Repair
Modification	Modification
Adjustment	Adjustment
Relabeling	Relabeling
Destruction	Destruction
Inspection	Inspection

error issue. Examples of the kinds of problems encountered with medical devices can be found on the FDA web page, "MedWatch Safety Alerts for Human Medical Products," at:

http://www.fda.gov/Safety/MedWatch/SafetyInformation/
SafetyAlertsforHumanMedicalProducts/default.htm

This page is an agency-level publication and contains links to alerts for all regulated products by year of issuance. Medical devices appear in a separate list under the year of choice. Each alert contains links to any associated recall notice and press release.

Section 2. Market Withdrawal versus Recall

Any particular correction or removal may constitute either a "market withdrawal" or a "recall." There are significant differences between these categories that affect the manufacturer's responsibilities and FDA's involvement in the process. Thus, it is important to distinguish between a "market withdrawal" of a device and a device "recall."

Market Withdrawals

A manufacturer generally makes the initial decision on whether a correction or removal constitutes a market withdrawal or a recall. Market withdrawals usually do not involve the device's safety or effectiveness, and the problems precipitating the action do not pose a risk of injury or illness to the user or patient. These kinds of problems may relate to marketing issues, customer satisfaction, convenience of use, and so on. In this case, the FDA does not have to be involved, and the manufacturer would service its customers in the normal course of business.

Recalls

If a manufacturer determines that it is dealing with a violative product, that is, the product is adulterated or misbranded, or the company is in violation of the QSR or other sections of the FDCA or regulations, the correction or removal of the device would constitute a recall. When the manufacturer identifies and initiates a recall, it would be a voluntary recall, discussed in section 4 below.

Section 3. Recall Classification

The agency classifies each recall action based on the risk to health posed by the defect. The risk to health is based on an examination of appropriate precedents within the agency's files or based on the outcome of a Health Hazard Evaluation (HHE). HHEs are discussed in section 5 below.

The recall classes are distinguished by the probability and severity of the risk. The classification of a recall will determine the urgency, depth, and extent of the recall. Each recall is classified into one of the following three classes:

- *Class I.* There is a *reasonable probability* that the use of or exposure to the violative product will cause serious adverse health consequences or death.

- *Class II.* The use of or exposure to the violative product *may cause* temporary or medically reversible adverse health consequences, or the probability of serious adverse health consequences is remote.

- *Class III.* The use of or exposure to the violative product is *not likely* to cause adverse health consequences.

Section 4. Voluntary Recalls

A firm may decide of its own volition and under any circumstances to remove or correct a distributed product. As stated above, if the device is regarded to be a violative product, the action would be considered a recall. Recalls of medical devices are voluntary unless mandated by FDA. Mandatory recalls are discussed in section 5 below.

Initiating a Voluntary Recall

Addressing post-market device problems is the responsibility of the firm. The vast majority of recalls are voluntary actions taken by the manufacturer. Typically, a firm recognizes a problem and takes appropriate corrective action. Alternatively, FDA may recognize a problem and request, as opposed to mandate, the manufacturer to undertake a recall. An order to conduct a mandatory recall is a last resort, but the agency will not hesitate to issue such an order if the hazard presented warrants such action.

Firm Responsibilities in Recalls

Even though a recall may be voluntarily conducted, the manufacturer has responsibilities that must be met. The firm must, in the first instance, determine the need for a recall. It must then conduct a risk assessment, determine the root cause of the problem, notify the FDA District Office, execute appropriate recall actions, and improve product quality for the future. Frequently, these actions by the manufacturer will take the form of a corrective and preventive action as specified in the Quality System Regulation and discussed in Chapter 7, part 8, Corrective and Preventive Actions.

Reporting Recall Actions to FDA

A firm must notify the FDA District Office for correction and removal of marketed products to discuss its strategy. The firm must report the action it takes to correct the problem or remove the device to FDA within 10 days of initiation of the action. The district recall coordinator alerts CDRH and collects more information. The FDA District Office prepares a package with recommendations for the Center to consider.

District Office Responsibilities in Recalls

The District Office has the following responsibilities during a recall:

- Provide regulatory oversight
- Comment on the firm's strategy
- Review the firm's communications
- Audit the effectiveness of the recall
- Witness product destruction or approve a reconditioning plan
- Determine compliance with 510(k) or PMA requirements
- Determine if the firm's action meets the definition of a recall
- Confirm recall precedents

CDRH Responsibilities

CDRH responsibilities include the following actions:

- Provide scientific and regulatory input to the district and the firm
- Assess the risk of the defect or the device failure
- Conduct a Health Hazard Evaluation
- Review company "Dear Dr." letters and press releases
- Classify the recall
- Prepare FDA press releases and public health notices

Section 5. Mandatory Recalls

When FDA becomes aware of a correction or removal of a medical device by the manufacturer, the agency may have a different opinion from the manufacturer on whether the action is a market withdrawal or a recall. In such a case, FDA may request the manufacturer to conduct a recall of the product. Most of the time, the manufacturer will comply with such a request from the FDA. In other instances, the FDA may become aware of a problem with a marketed device through its own surveillance of the marketplace and from its own information sources. In such a case, the FDA may likewise request a recall by the manufacturer.

In either of the foregoing cases, if the manufacturer does not comply, FDA may order the manufacturer to institute a mandatory recall. FDA can mandate a recall based on risk of illness or injury and/or gross consumer deception.

Determination of Risk

FDA will determine the extent of the risk presented by the device defect involved in the recall. As a first step, CDRH will examine past decisions in similar cases. The Center will look at its precedents files for similar product experiences, similar problems of device failures, and similar risks to health. A medical officer reviews the precedents to assure that they are appropriate to the device, failure mode, population, and intended use under consideration. If no appropriate precedent is found, the Center may conduct a Health Hazard Evaluation.

Health Hazard Evaluation

A Health Hazard Evaluation is a formal, regulatory-based risk assessment following established procedures to guide the Center in classifying a recall and determining what actions are needed by the firm and FDA to protect the public health. A separate assessment is conducted for each type of device or failure mode involved. The HHE becomes part of FDA's long-term files. It provides a precedent, if applicable, for future recalls and supports later enforcement actions. It may also be used in legal proceedings.

The form requires an identification and analysis of the problem and reason for the recall, the findings of the manufacturer's CAPA investigation, and an evaluation of the immediate and long-range health consequences of the device failure. The HHE form can be found at:

http://www.fda.gov/MedicalDevices/DeviceRegulationand
Guidance/IVDRegulatoryAssistance/ucm126206.htm

In addition to the lack of an appropriate precedent, an HHE may be conducted if the risk appears high and a recall is likely to be a Class I or Class II recall, or if the recall presents a unique scientific, clinical, or public health issue.

The HHE is conducted by a medical officer and others as needed. The evaluation will identify the population at risk, the conditions that may increase or reduce the risk of the hazard's occurrence, the risk associated with the product under labeled conditions of use, and the likelihood of the risk occurring in the future.

The HHE is based on currently available information and may be updated as the situation unfolds. It may incorporate information from the manufacturer, premarket submissions, MDRs, complaints by users, scientific information, and the professional and scientific literature.

During the HHE, some of the factors that will be considered include:

- Whether injuries have already occurred

- Whether the problem is easily detectable by the user

- Existing conditions that could expose users to a health hazard

- The hazard posed to the population at greatest risk

- The severity of the hazard

- The likelihood of occurrence of the hazard

- The immediate and long-range health consequences

Once an HHE is completed, it may be used as a guide for the recall strategy, including letters and press releases by the firm. Beyond the recall, the HHE may help evaluate the firm's quality systems, guide any FDA outreach to providers and patients, guide FDA priorities and workload related to the types of devices or defects involved, and guide actions taken by other firms.

Section 6. Managing Recalls

The agency's role during a recall is to review and guide the firm conducting the recall. FDA monitors the process to assure that the fix is appropriate. The agency has established very short time frames, often only hours or days, for recall activities, the time depending on the level of risk to individuals.

FDA's District Offices have the primary role in monitoring a recall, and CDRH offices may assist and provide expertise as needed. The Center works with the District Office and the firm to assure that the public health is protected by confirming that the recall strategy clearly communicates the risk to device users and patients, assessing the firm's plan to monitor the recall, and conducting a final audit check.

Beyond the recall, CDRH evaluates the firm's quality system to determine whether the corrective and preventive action process was sufficient, the root cause of the problem was fixed, and a validation was conducted when the fix was implemented. CDRH will not concur with the termination of the recall until the corrective action has been validated.

Termination of a Recall

A recall will be terminated when the Food and Drug Administration determines that all reasonable efforts have been made to remove or correct the product in accordance with the recall strategy, and when it is reasonable to assume that the product subject to the recall has been removed and proper disposition or correction has been made commensurate with the degree of hazard presented by the recalled product.

Other FDA Actions

Depending on the severity and cause of the defects underlying a recall, FDA may take additional compliance actions. Generally, such a product will be adulterated or misbranded, the company may be in violation of the QSR regulations, or there may be other violations of the act or regulations. These violations may result in fines or other penalties, which are outlined in Chapter 8, Compliance and Enforcement.

Section 7. Examples of Medical Device Recalls

Recalls are, unfortunately, regular and sometimes frequent occurrences in the medical device industry. There are many reasons why recalls have to be initiated, as discussed in the above sections. They may be related to any aspect of medical device design, testing, manufacture, labeling, packaging, and so on. FDA wastes no time in publishing information that a recall has occurred and the basis for the recall because of the risk of harm that may be presented by a recalled medical device. In addition to any other form of notification that may be used by the manufacturer or FDA, the agency posts information about serious recalls within 24 hours of the classification of a recall. In addition to the FDA recall pages cited above, the agency maintains a searchable database of medical device recalls at:

> http://www.accessdata.fda.gov/scripts/cdrh/cfdocs/cfRES/
> res.cfm

Below are four representative selections from the recall information posted on the FDA website. The information is frequently provided by the firm conducting the recall, and further information may be available from the recalling manufacturer. These examples illustrate the variety of causes underlying the need for a recall.

Electrical Board Short Circuit

> Physio-Control, Inc., a division of Medtronic, Inc., is conducting a voluntary correction for a limited number of LIFEPAK 15 monitor/

defibrillators. Our internal analysis has verified that for those monitor/defibrillators an internal component could inadvertently contact the power printed circuit board assembly (PCBA). Should this occur, we have verified that the monitor/defibrillator may:

- cycle power Off then On by itself, or
- power Off by itself requiring the operator to turn it back On, or
- stay powered On and not allow itself to be turned Off.

Pin Holes in Sterile IV Tubing Set Packaging

Testing of the Teleflex Incorporated–Arrow International Custom Intravenous (IV) Administration Products (IV Tubing Sets and Accessories) and Certain Arrow Arterial Embolectomy Catheters revealed pinholes or punctures in the sterile Tyvek packaging. Because of these defects, the products may no longer be sterile. This may potentially cause blood-borne or other types of infections, which could result in serious injury or death.

Surgical Computer Workstation Failure

The Stryker Corporation Operating Room System II Surgical Navigation Systems may suddenly stop working, the screen may freeze, or the information may only be updated very slowly. These problems may affect all software products. These failures could result in delay in surgery, rescheduling of the procedure resulting in an additional surgery, risk of infection, increased disease symptoms, potential neurological problems, or injury due to the surgeon operating in an area where they did not intend to operate. Depending on the type of surgery, these failures could potentially lead to serious adverse health consequences, including death.

Implanted Vertebral Body Integrity Failure

The Synthes Ti Synex II Vertebral Body Replacement (VBR) was the subject of adverse events reports that included moderate to severe loss of vertebral body replacement height (caused by failure of the central body component) in situ at six to fifteen months post implantation. Potential adverse health issues that could be associated with this issue include neural injury, increased pain, spinal kyphosis if unrecognized, failure of supplementary fixation, and/or need for reoperation/revision surgery.

PART 5. NOTIFICATION AND THREE R's

Requiring notification, repair, replacement, and refund constitute additional means for FDA to deal with violative products. They offer FDA a way of requiring a manufacturer to notify users of fraudulent, defective, or otherwise hazardous products, and provide the agency with the tools to assure that hazardous products in the hands of consumers and other users are repaired, replaced, or refunded. In addition to the public health purpose of these actions, they also give consumers a procedure for economic redress when they have been sold defective medical devices that present unreasonable risks.

It can be noted that a consumer of a defective device may have non-FDA recourse for redress under contract law or commercial law if the device is not "fungible" or "suitable for a particular purpose." A consumer may also have a cause of action under the law of negligence or product liability for injuries incurred by the use of the device. These actions are outside the purview of this book and are not discussed.

Section 1. Notification

FDA may require manufacturers or other appropriate individuals to notify all health professionals who prescribe or use the device, and any other person (including manufacturers, importers, distributors, retailers, and device users), of the health risks resulting from the use of the violative device so that these risks may be reduced or eliminated.

Threshold Requirements

FDA can order notification if a device presents an unreasonable risk of substantial harm to public health, notification is necessary to eliminate the risk, and no more practicable means are available under the FDCA to eliminate the risk.

Procedures

The procedures for a notification order are simple. They involve only prior consultation with the persons who are to provide the notification.

Section 2. Repair, Replacement, or Refund (Three R's)

FDA may, after offering an opportunity for an informal hearing, order manufacturers, importers, or distributors to repair, replace, or refund the purchase price of devices that present unreasonable health risks.

Basic Criteria

The FDA can order repair, replacement, or refund if, after the opportunity for an informal hearing, it determines that:

- The device represents an unreasonable risk of substantial harm to the public health

- The device was not designed and manufactured in accordance with the then-prevailing state of the art

- The risk is not due to negligent installation, maintenance, repair, or use of the device by persons other than a manufacturer, importer, distributor, or retailer, and

- Notification alone is insufficient, and repair, replacement, or refund is necessary

Procedures

The procedures for repair, replacement, or refund are complex and could result in multiple orders, regulatory hearings, and many delays if FDA and the manufacturer, or other responsible person, are unable to agree on a plan for addressing a risk. The agency must consider available alternatives. Both notification orders and repair, replacement, or refund orders are discretionary. Before ordering notification, FDA must determine that no more practical means are available under the FDCA to eliminate the risk. Although there is no requirement that such a determination be made before FDA orders repair, replacement, or refund, FDA must determine that notification alone is insufficient before ordering repair, replacement, or refund.

There are several alternatives available to FDA under these circumstances. FDA may institute a legal action such as seizure, injunction, or prosecutions. FDA may promulgate a rule such as banning the device or imposing restrictions on sale, distribution, or use. The agency may also order a recall, which is discussed above in part 4, Medical Device Recalls.

PART 6. EXERCISES

1. What is the purpose of the Medical Device Reporting program, and what are reportable events?

2. What constitutes (1) a serious illness or injury and (2) a device malfunction or failure?

3. Search FDA's MDR database and identify a report that involved a death, one that included a serious injury, and one that included

a device malfunction. For each report, identify the name of the device, the name of the manufacturer, the device defect, and the effect of the defect.

4. When and how may FDA order the conduct of a post-market surveillance study?

5. Search the FDA post-market surveillance database. Select and describe a PS study that involves a public health concern resulting from reported or suspected problems in a marketed device.

6. Describe how the medical tracking process works.

7. What actions by a manufacturer constitute a device correction or removal, and what are the bases for such an action?

8. When a manufacturer makes a correction or removal of a medical device, how does one determine whether the action is a withdrawal or a recall, and what are the consequences of either one?

9. How are recalls classified?

10. What is a Health Hazard Evaluation, and how is it conducted?

11. Search the FDA recall database and identify three recall notices that represent a design failure, a materials failure, and a durability failure. For each recall, identify the device, the manufacturer, the date, and the device defect. Explain how the defect presents a health hazard and what can be done to correct the problem.

7

Quality Systems and GMPs

OVERVIEW

The main requirements that apply to the manufacturing aspects of medical devices are set forth in the Quality System Regulation (QSR). The current QSR was promulgated on November 7, 1996, and it has been amended several times since then. It supplanted, and incorporated, the previous requirements referred to as Current Good Manufacturing Practices or cGMPs.

A major change to the previous cGMP regulation was the addition of design controls, including human factors engineering, which are discussed in Chapter 2, Medical Device Design. This chapter deals with the remaining elements of the QSR dealing primarily with the GMP aspects of manufacturing.

The QSR is complex and detailed. This chapter provides an overview of the QSR requirements. For those who are interested in a more detailed and expanded discussion of the QSR regulatory requirements, there are books devoted to the subject, including international quality system requirements, as well as courses provided by specialists in the field.

It should also be pointed out that the QSR requirements represent a minimum baseline for an effective quality assurance program. Many companies have sophisticated quality assurance programs that go beyond the QSR requirements based on the particular needs of their operations and the devices they produce.

APPLICABILITY OF QSR

The QSR states that these requirements "govern the methods used in, and the facilities and controls used for, the design, manufacture, packaging, labeling, storage, installation, and servicing of all finished devices intended for human use."

One of the ultimate purposes of the QSR is to assure that marketed devices will be quality products that are safe and effective and in compliance with the law. It applies to devices manufactured in, imported, or offered for import into the United States or Puerto Rico.

Unless they are subject to premarket review under the device provisions of the FDCA or biological license requirements of the Public Health Service Act, the QSR does not apply to:

- Manufacturers of components or parts

- Manufacturers of blood and blood components

- Manufacturers of human cells, tissues, and cellular and tissue-based products

MEDICAL DEVICE QUALITY

The primary goal and objective to be achieved in the manufacture of a medical device is to produce a quality product. A quality product, as opposed to an inferior or defective product, provides greater assurance that the mass-produced device will perform as planned and be as safe and effective as possible. Therefore, a short description of "quality" is appropriate, if not essential, as a precursor to a discussion of the Quality System Regulation.

The meaning of "quality" has been extensively discussed and debated in the literature, and there are many variations on the topic. Here are some interesting ideas on the meaning of quality and related matters:

Quality in business, engineering, and manufacturing has a pragmatic interpretation as the non-inferiority or superiority of something. Quality is a perceptual, conditional, and somewhat subjective attribute, and may be understood differently by different people. Consumers may focus on the specification quality of a product/service, or how it compares to competitors in the marketplace. Producers might measure the conformance quality, or degree to which the product/service was produced correctly.

Numerous definitions and methodologies have been created to assist in managing the quality-affecting aspects of business operations. Many different techniques and concepts have evolved to improve product or service quality. There are two common quality-related functions within a business. One is quality assurance, which is the prevention of defects, such as by the deployment of a quality management system and preventive activities like FMEA. The other is quality control, which is the detection of defects, most commonly associated with testing which takes place within a quality management system, typically referred to as verification and validation.

The common element of the business definitions is that the quality of a product or service refers to the perception of the degree to which the product or service meets the customer's expectations. Quality has no specific meaning unless related to a specific function and/or object. Quality is a perceptual, conditional, and somewhat subjective attribute.

The business meanings of quality have developed over time. Various interpretations are given below:

1. ISO 9000: "Degree to which a set of inherent characteristics fulfills requirements." The standard defines requirement as need or expectation.

   . . .

9. American Society for Quality: "A subjective term for which each person has his or her own definition. In technical usage, quality can have two meanings:

   a. The characteristics of a product or service that bear on its ability to satisfy stated or implied needs;

   b. A product or service free of deficiencies."

10. Peter Drucker: "Quality in a product or service is not what the supplier puts in. It is what the customer gets out and is willing to pay for."

11. W. Edwards Deming: concentrating on "the efficient production of the quality that the market expects," and he linked quality and management: "Costs go down and productivity goes up as improvement of quality is accomplished by better management of design, engineering, testing and by improvement of processes."

The excerpts quoted above are taken from an extensive article on the topic of quality at:

http://en.wikipedia.org/wiki/Quality_(business)

MANUFACTURER FUNCTIONS TO ASSURE THE QUALITY OF MEDICAL DEVICES

There are many ways in which manufacturers can provide greater assurance that the medical devices they design and manufacture are of the highest quality possible. Listed below are just some of the major principles they may adopt and implement to assure the quality of their products. Most of these principles are, in fact, required by FDA and are discussed throughout this book.

- Develop an effective design control plan

- Conduct risk analyses

- Follow adequate and appropriate SOPs/protocols for nonclinical and clinical testing

- Monitor and audit clinical trials

- Establish and implement a company-wide quality policy

- Conduct quality audits

- Implement a quality control program

- Maintain, analyze, and follow up on complaint files

- Adopt and implement, when necessary, a corrective and preventive action plan

ELEMENTS OF QSR/GMPs

This chapter deals with the QSR with the exception of design control, which, as stated above, is discussed in Chapter 2, Medical Device Design. This chapter covers the remaining areas of the QSR requirements and QSIT inspections under the following subjects:

- Management and organization—Part 1

- Document controls—Part 2

- Purchasing controls—Part 3

- Identification and traceability—Part 4

- Production and process controls—Part 5

- Acceptance activities—Part 6

- Nonconforming product—Part 7

- Corrective and preventive actions—Part 8

- Labeling and packaging controls—Part 9

- Handling, storage, distribution, and installation—Part 10

- Records—Part 11

- Servicing and statistical techniques—Part 12

- QSIT inspections—Part 13

PART 1. MANAGEMENT AND ORGANIZATION

Section 1. Management Responsibilities

General Responsibilities

A firm's management has responsibilities in three major areas of medical device manufacturing: (1) integrity of various organizational functions, (2) managing the quality audit process, and (3) personnel responsibilities. More specifically, management has the responsibility to ensure the integrity of: the quality policy, organizational structure, in-house responsibilities and authorities, resources, management's representative, reporting to management, quality audit activities, and personnel.

Responsibility for Quality

Management with executive responsibility must undertake the following actions in order to satisfactorily discharge its duty concerning quality within the firm:

- Quality system policy

    - Management must establish the company policy and objectives for, and commitment to, quality.

    - It must ensure that the quality policy is understood, implemented, and maintained at all levels of the organization.

- Quality system procedures

  - Manufacturers must establish quality system procedures and instructions.

  - An outline of the structure of the documentation used in the quality system must be established where appropriate.

- Quality planning

  - Manufacturers have to establish a quality plan that defines the quality practices, resources, and activities relevant to devices that are designed and manufactured.

  - The manufacturer must establish how the requirements for quality will be met.

- Quality audit

  - To assure that the quality system is in compliance with the established quality system requirements and to determine the effectiveness of the quality system, manufacturers must:

    - Establish procedures for quality audits

    - Conduct such audits

  - Quality audits are to be conducted by individuals who do not have direct responsibility for the matters being audited.

  - Corrective actions, including a reaudit of deficient matters, must be taken when deficiencies are found.

  - At the conclusion of each quality audit and reaudit:

    - The auditor has to make a report of the results of the audit.

    - Management having responsibility for the matters audited must review the audit report.

  - The dates and results of quality audits and reaudits must be documented.

- Management review

  - Management with executive responsibility must review the suitability and effectiveness of the quality system at defined intervals and with sufficient frequency, according to established procedures, to ensure that the quality system satisfies the requirements of the manufacturer's established quality policy and objectives.

- The dates and results of quality system reviews must be documented.

Section 2. Organization

Manufacturers must have three elements for an adequate organizational structure to ensure that devices are designed and produced in accordance with QSR:

- *Responsibility and authority.* There must be appropriate responsibility, authority, and interrelation of all personnel who manage, perform, and assess work affecting quality, and the independence and authority necessary to perform these tasks must be provided.

- *Resources.* There need to be adequate resources, including the assignment of trained personnel, for management, performance of work, and assessment activities, including internal quality audits.

- *Management representative.* The company needs to appoint, and document such appointment of, a member of management who has established authority over and responsibility for:

  - Ensuring that quality system requirements are effectively established and effectively maintained

  - Reporting on the performance of the quality system to management with executive responsibility for review

Section 3. Personnel

Manufacturers have to have sufficient personnel with the necessary education, background, training, and experience to assure that all activities required by the regulations are correctly performed. There must be procedures for identifying training needs, and training to ensure that all personnel can adequately perform their assigned responsibilities.

As part of their training, personnel must be made aware of device defects that might occur from the improper performance of their specific jobs, and their training must be documented.

Lastly, personnel who perform verification and validation activities need to be made aware of defects and errors that may be encountered as part of their job functions.

PART 2. DOCUMENT CONTROLS

General Requirement

Each manufacturer must establish and maintain procedures to control all documents required under the QSR. This includes both original documents and changes to documents.

Section 1. Document Approval and Distribution

This section of the QSR deals with three elements of document control and distribution: document creation, approving individual, and document distribution. A designated individual must review for adequacy and approve all documents established to meet the regulatory requirements prior to issuance. The approval, including the date and signature of the individual approving the document, must be documented. Documents established to meet the requirements of QSR must be made available at all locations for which they are designated, used, or are otherwise necessary. Obsolete documents have to be promptly removed from all points of use or otherwise prevented from unintended use.

Section 2. Document Changes

Changes to documents are reviewed and approved by an individual in the same function or organization that performed the original review and approval, unless specifically designated otherwise. Approved changes must be communicated to the appropriate personnel in a timely manner, and each manufacturer must maintain records of changes to documents. Change records must include:

- A description of the change
- Identification of the affected documents
- The signature of the approving individual

- The approval date
- The effective date

PART 3. PURCHASING CONTROLS

General Requirement

Each manufacturer must establish and maintain procedures to ensure that all purchased or otherwise received products and services conform to specified requirements.

Section 1. Evaluation of Suppliers, Contractors, and Consultants

Each manufacturer has to establish and maintain the requirements, including quality requirements, that must be met by suppliers, contractors, and consultants. They must:

- Evaluate and select potential suppliers, contractors, and consultants on the basis of their ability to meet specified requirements, including quality requirements and regulatory requirements. The evaluations must be documented.

- Define the type and extent of control to be exercised over the product, services, suppliers, contractors, and consultants, based on the evaluation results.

- Establish and maintain records of acceptable suppliers, contractors, and consultants.

More and more manufacturers are incorporating into the purchase contract the right to inspect, monitor, and audit the facilities and operations of the suppliers, as well as their products, to ensure that the products will meet the purchaser's quality requirements and applicable regulatory requirements. This is especially important in the age of the global market and multiple sources of supply. In response to this need, the FDA is enhancing the training of its investigators to identify weaknesses in this area and the GHTF has issued a guidance that includes the auditing of manufacturers' purchasing controls.

Section 2. Purchasing Data

Each medical device manufacturer must establish and maintain data that clearly describe or reference the specified requirements, including quality requirements, for purchased or otherwise received products and services.

The purchasing documents should include, where possible, an agreement that the suppliers, contractors, and consultants will notify the manufacturer of changes in the product, its materials or components, and service so that manufacturers may determine whether the changes might affect the quality of a finished device, and continue to meet the specifications of the purchaser.

Purchasing data must comply with document controls.

PART 4. IDENTIFICATION AND TRACEABILITY

Section 1. Identification

Each manufacturer must establish and maintain procedures for identifying products during all stages of receipt, production, distribution, and installation to prevent mix-ups.

Section 2. Traceability

Each manufacturer must establish and maintain procedures for identifying with a control number each unit, lot, or batch of finished devices that is intended:

- For surgical implant into the body, or

- To support or sustain life, and

- Whose failure to perform when properly used in accordance with instructions for use provided in the labeling can be reasonably expected to result in a significant injury to the user

These procedures must include, where appropriate, components of a device.

Such identification needs to be documented in the device history record (DHR), as discussed below in part 11, Records.

These procedures should facilitate corrective actions, which are discussed below in part 8, Corrective and Preventive Actions. This traceability requirement also ties in directly with the discussion in Chapter 6, part 3, Medical Device Tracking.

PART 5. PRODUCTION AND PROCESS CONTROLS

General Requirement

QSR requires manufacturers to develop, conduct, control, and monitor production processes to ensure that a device conforms to its specifications. Where deviations from device specifications could occur as a result of the manufacturing process, there must be process control procedures that describe any process controls necessary to ensure conformance to specifications.

While the QSR deals with manufacturing, it is interesting to note the similarities in the requirements related to production and process controls and the controls required for device design as presented in Chapter 2, Medical Device Design, and in the area of laboratory practices as discussed in Chapter 3, Nonclinical Testing and GLPs.

Section 1. Production and Process Controls

The manufacturer must prepare and maintain documented instructions, standard operating procedures (SOPs), and methods that define and control the manner of production. These SOPs should include, at least, the following topics:

- Monitoring and control of process parameters and component and device characteristics during production

- Compliance with specified reference standards or codes

- The approval of processes and process equipment

- Criteria for workmanship, which shall be expressed in documented standards or by means of identified and approved representative samples

Section 2. Areas of Control

The production and processing of medical devices that require control can be broken down into the following five areas.

Production and Process Changes

The manufacturer must establish and maintain procedures for changes to a specification, method, process, or procedure. Such changes need to be verified and/or validated in accordance with process validation requirements before implementation. As in so many other cases, these activities require documentation and approval in accordance with document control requirements.

Environmental Control

Where environmental conditions could reasonably be expected to have an adverse effect on product quality, the manufacturer must establish and maintain procedures to adequately control these environmental conditions. Environmental control systems have to be periodically inspected to verify that the system and necessary equipment are adequate and functioning properly. Documentation and review are necessary.

Personnel

Manufacturers must have requirements for the health, cleanliness, personal practices, and clothing of personnel if contact between such personnel and product or environment could reasonably be expected to have an adverse effect on product quality.

The manufacturer must ensure that maintenance and other personnel who are required to work temporarily under special environmental conditions are appropriately trained or supervised by a trained individual.

Contamination Control

Procedures are required to prevent contamination of equipment or product by substances that could reasonably be expected to have an adverse effect on product quality.

Buildings

Buildings must be of suitable design and contain sufficient space to perform necessary operations, prevent mix-ups, and assure orderly handling.

Section 3. Equipment Controls

All equipment used in the manufacturing process must meet specified requirements and be appropriately designed, constructed, placed, and installed to facilitate maintenance, adjustment, cleaning, and use. Each manufacturer must also establish and maintain schedules for the adjustment, cleaning, and other maintenance of equipment to ensure that manufacturing specifications are met. Maintenance activities must be documented, including the date and the names of the individuals performing the tasks.

Equipment Calibration

Equipment calibration has come under recent scrutiny by FDA because the agency has seen that companies are blindly accepting calibration certificates from test houses. Test houses are third parties used by firms to ensure that equipment used in the manufacture or the inspection and testing of their devices is properly calibrated and maintained.

When a test house returns a report that indicates a piece of equipment had been out of specification, it is incumbent on the manufacturer to review the product manufactured with or tested with the equipment that had been out of specification. It is important to confirm that the equipment in question did not have an adverse effect on devices already manufactured. If it did, corrective actions would be indicated.

Appropriate purchasing contracts, as discussed in part 3 above, that include monitoring, auditing, and inspection of the supplier, in this case a testing house, can provide assurance that the testing was conducted appropriately for the needs of the purchaser.

PART 6. ACCEPTANCE ACTIVITIES

General Requirement

Manufacturers must have procedures for acceptance activities, which include inspections, tests, and other verification activities.

Section 1. Inspection and Adjustment

Periodic inspections as required by established procedures to ensure adherence to applicable equipment maintenance schedules need to be documented, including the date and individuals conducting the inspections.

Any inherent limitations or allowable tolerances must be visibly posted on or near equipment requiring periodic adjustments, or must be readily available to personnel performing these adjustments.

Section 2. Receiving and In-Process Acceptance

The established procedures must also include procedures for acceptance of incoming product. Incoming product must be inspected, tested, or otherwise verified as conforming to specified requirements, and acceptance or rejection must be documented. In addition, acceptance procedures are required to ensure that specified requirements for in-process product are met.

Such procedures are to ensure that in-process product is controlled until the required inspection and tests or other verification activities have been completed, or necessary approvals are received and documented.

Section 3. Final Acceptance and Records

Final Acceptance

Final acceptance activities include the following:

- Each manufacturer must establish and maintain procedures for finished device acceptance to ensure that each production run, lot, or batch of finished devices meets acceptance criteria.

- Finished devices have to be held in quarantine or otherwise adequately controlled until released.

- Finished devices may not be released for distribution until:

  – The activities required in the device master record (DMR), discussed below in part 11, Records, are completed

  – The associated data and documentation are reviewed

  – The release is authorized by the signature of a designated individual(s)

  – The authorization is dated

Acceptance Records

Each manufacturer must document acceptance activities required under QSR. These records must include:

- The acceptance activities performed

- The dates on which acceptance activities are performed

- The results

- The signature of the individual(s) conducting the acceptance activities

- Where appropriate, the equipment used

- Making the records part of the DHR

PART 7. NONCONFORMING PRODUCT

The QSR requires procedures to control product that does not conform to specified requirements. These procedures should address the identification and evaluation of the nonconforming product, its segregation and disposition, and the documentation of these activities.

The evaluation must include a determination of the need for an investigation, and notification of the persons or organizations responsible for the nonconformance. The evaluation and investigation need to be documented.

The procedures for dealing with nonconforming products must specify who is responsible for reviewing the nonconforming product, who has the authority for its disposition, and what the review and disposition process is.

There must be procedures that cover rework of nonconforming product, including its retesting and reevaluation after rework, ensuring that the product meets its current approved specifications, and that the rework and reevaluation activities, including a determination of any adverse effect from the rework of the product, are documented in the DHR.

Documentation for the disposition of nonconforming product should include the justification for use of nonconforming product and the signature of the individual authorizing the use.

PART 8. CORRECTIVE AND PREVENTIVE ACTIONS

General Requirement

Manufacturers need procedures to identify existing and potential causes of nonconforming product or other quality problems and for implementing corrective and preventive actions (CAPAs).

It should be pointed out at this time that these CAPA principles and procedures are not just applicable in dealing with manufacturing process problems. These principles are applicable under any circumstances in which a corrective and preventive action is required whether related to design, testing, premarket, or post-market problems. See, for example, the discussions in Chapter 6, Post-Market Responsibilities, and Chapter 8, Compliance and Enforcement. CAPA principles also are applicable under an AIP/IH action as discussed in Chapter 5, part 1, section 8, Data Integrity.

There are a series of steps identified in the QSR that are required to assure that an acceptable corrective and preventive action plan is adopted and implemented.

Section 1. Analysis of the Problem

The QSR requires the audit and analysis of any of the following items, as applicable:

- Processes
- Work operations
- Concessions
- Quality audit reports
- Quality records
- Service records
- Complaints
- Returned product
- Other sources of quality data

In conducting a quality audit and analysis, appropriate statistical methodology should be employed to detect recurring quality problems with product, processes, and the quality system. The audit and analysis should identify the actions needed to correct and prevent recurrence of nonconforming products and other quality problems.

In the area of AIP/IH, complete system and data auditing is necessary to identify the cause of the unreliability of the records, including the identification of any individuals that may be responsible for the data errors, to verify the accuracy and completeness of data and information submitted in the application, and to construct appropriate corrective and preventive actions.

Different types of auditing are dealt with in Chapter 1, part 11, Monitoring and Auditing.

Section 2. Other Actions

In addition to a quality audit and analysis of the problem, the following actions must be taken:

- Verifying or validating the corrective and preventive action necessary to ensure that such action is effective and does not adversely affect the finished device.

- Ensuring that information is disseminated to those directly responsible for assuring the quality of such product, or the prevention of such problems, if necessary.

- Relevant information on identified quality problems, as well as corrective and preventive actions, must be submitted for management review.

- The process should result in implementing and recording changes in methods and procedures needed to correct and prevent identified quality problems.

All of these activities must be documented.

PART 9. LABELING AND PACKAGING CONTROLS

Section 1. Labeling

Labels have to remain legible and affixed during the customary conditions of processing, storage, handling, distribution, and use of the device. Labeling is not to be released for storage or use until a designated individual has examined the labeling for accuracy, including the expiration date, control number, storage instructions, handling instructions, and processing instructions.

The release, including the date and signature of the individuals performing the examination, must be documented in the DHR. The DHR is explained below in part 11, Records.

Labeling has to be stored in a manner that provides proper identification and is designed to prevent mix-ups. Manufacturers need to control labeling and packaging operations to prevent labeling mix-ups.

The label and labeling used for each production unit, lot, or batch must be documented in the DHR. Where a control number is required for purposes of traceability, that control number must be on or shall accompany the device through distribution. The requirement for control numbers and other identifications is discussed above in part 4, Identification and Traceability.

Section 2. Packaging

The manufacturer has to ensure that device packaging and shipping containers are designed and constructed to protect the device from alteration or damage during the customary conditions of processing, storage, handling, and distribution.

PART 10. HANDLING, STORAGE, DISTRIBUTION, AND INSTALLATION

Section 1. Handling and Storage

Manufacturers must have procedures to ensure that:

- Mix-up, damage, deterioration, contamination, or other adverse effects to product do not occur during handling.

- No obsolete, rejected, or deteriorated product is used or distributed.

- Control is maintained over storage areas and stock rooms.

- Product is stored to facilitate proper stock rotation and so that its condition is assessed, as appropriate.

They also need procedures that describe the methods for authorizing receipt from and dispatch to storage areas and stock rooms.

Section 2. Distribution

Procedures for control and distribution of finished devices must ensure that only those devices approved for release are distributed and that purchase orders are reviewed to ensure that ambiguities and errors are resolved before devices are released for distribution. The procedures have to ensure that expired devices or devices deteriorated beyond acceptable fitness for use are not distributed. Distribution records have to include or refer to the location of:

- The name and address of the initial consignee

- The identification and quantity of devices shipped

- The date shipped

- Any control numbers used

Section 3. Installation

When a device requires installation, the manufacturer must have instructions and directions for installation, inspection, and test procedures. The instructions and procedures must accompany the device, or they have to be made available to those installing the device. The person installing the device has to ensure that the installation, inspection, and any required testing are performed in accordance with the manufacturer's instructions and procedures and that the documentation of the inspection and test results demonstrate proper installation.

PART 11. RECORDS

This part deals with the QSR record-keeping requirements. These requirements represent the general obligations of all manufacturers concerning the maintenance of adequate and readily available records. However, there are some specific activities that a manufacturer may engage in that carry with them additional record-keeping requirements that are unique to the specific activity. Manufacturers must comply with these specific record-keeping requirements. These other record-keeping requirements are discussed throughout this book in relation to the activities to which they apply. See, for example, Chapter 6, part 1, Medical Device Reporting.

Section 1. General Requirements

All QSR records shall be maintained at the manufacturing establishment or other location that is reasonably accessible to responsible officials of the manufacturer and to employees of FDA. The records should meet the following standards:

- All records must be made readily available for review and copying by FDA employees.

- Records have to be legible and stored to minimize deterioration and to prevent loss.

- There must be backups for records stored in automated data processing systems.

- Records deemed confidential by the manufacturer may be marked to aid FDA in determining whether information may be disclosed under the public information regulation.

- All records under QSR should be retained for a period of time equivalent to the design time and expected life of the device, but in no case less than two years from the date of release for commercial distribution by the manufacturer.

Exception

This section does not apply to the reports required for management reviews and quality audits, discussed above in part 1, Management and Organization, or supplier evaluations and audits, per part 3, Purchasing Controls, unless these processes include procedures adopted under the QSR record-keeping requirements. To accommodate these exceptions, a management employee of the manufacturer with executive responsibility must, upon request of a designated employee of FDA, certify in writing that the management reviews and quality audits required under this part, and supplier audits where applicable, have been performed and documented, including the dates on which they were performed, and that any required corrective and preventive actions have been undertaken.

Section 2. Device Master Records

Each manufacturer must maintain device master records (DMRs) and ensure that each DMR is prepared and approved in accordance with document control requirements as discussed above in part 2, Document Controls. The DMR for *each type of device* has to include or identify the location of the following information:

- Device specifications, including appropriate drawings, composition, formulation, component specifications, and software specifications

- Production process specifications, including the appropriate equipment specifications, production methods, production procedures, and production environment specifications

- Quality assurance procedures and specifications, including acceptance criteria and the quality assurance equipment to be used

- Packaging and labeling specifications, including methods and processes used

- Installation, maintenance, and servicing procedures and methods

Section 3. Device History Records

Each manufacturer has to maintain device history records (DHRs) and establish and maintain procedures to ensure that DHRs for *each batch, lot, or unit* are maintained to demonstrate that the device is manufactured in accordance with the DMR and other requirements of QSR. The DHR must include or refer to the location of the following information:

- The dates of manufacture

- The quantity manufactured

- The quantity released for distribution

- The acceptance records that demonstrate that the device is manufactured in accordance with the DMR

- The primary identification label and labeling used for each production unit

- Any device identification and control numbers used

Section 4. Quality System Records

Each manufacturer shall maintain a *quality system record* (QR). The QR shall include or identify the location of procedures, and the documentation of activities, required by this part that are not specific to a particular type of device, including, but not limited to, the management responsibility records. Each manufacturer shall ensure that the QR is prepared and approved in accordance with document control requirements.

Section 5. Complaint Files

Each manufacturer must have procedures and files for evaluating and documenting complaints. This is very important because of the actions that may have to be taken in response to identified problems.

Complaint-Handling Procedures

Each manufacturer must establish and maintain procedures for receiving, reviewing, and evaluating complaints by a formally designated unit. The designated unit may be an in-house unit, an off-site unit, or another organization under contract for this purpose.

Such procedures shall ensure that all complaints are processed in a uniform and timely manner and that oral complaints are documented upon receipt. The procedures must also specify that complaints are evaluated to determine whether the complaint represents an event that is required to be reported to FDA as explained in Chapter 6, part 1, Medical Device Reporting.

Evaluation and Investigation of Complaints

When a complaint is received, the manufacturer has to review and evaluate it to determine whether an investigation is necessary. When no investigation is made, the manufacturer must maintain a record that includes the reason no investigation was made and the name of the individual responsible for the decision not to investigate. However, any complaint involving the possible failure of a device, labeling, or packaging to meet any of its specifications must be reviewed, evaluated, and investigated, unless such investigation has already been performed for a similar complaint and another investigation is not necessary.

When an investigation is made under this section, a record of the investigation needs to be maintained by the formally designated unit identified above. The record of investigation should include:

- The name of the device
- The date the complaint was received
- Any device identification and control numbers used
- The name, address, and phone number of the complainant
- The nature and details of the complaint
- The dates and results of the investigation
- Any corrective action taken
- Any reply to the complainant

In addition to the foregoing information, records of investigation under this paragraph should include a determination of:

- Whether the device failed to meet specifications
- Whether the device was being used for treatment or diagnosis
- The relationship, if any, of the device to the reported incident or adverse event

MDR Reporting to FDA

Any complaint that represents an event that must be reported to FDA under MDR must be promptly reviewed, evaluated, and investigated by a designated individual and maintained in a separate portion of the complaint files or in a separate MDR file. In either case it must be clearly identified as an MDR record. These events must also be reported to FDA under MDR.

Location of Records

When the manufacturer's formally designated complaint unit is located at a site separate from the manufacturing establishment, the investigated complaints and the records of investigation must be reasonably accessible to the manufacturing establishment.

If a manufacturer's formally designated complaint unit is located outside of the United States, records required by this section shall be reasonably accessible in the United States at either a location in the United States where the manufacturer's records are regularly kept or at the location of the initial distributor.

PART 12. SERVICING AND STATISTICAL TECHNIQUES

This part combines two distinct QSR requirements: servicing and statistical techniques.

Section 1. Servicing

Where servicing is a specified requirement, each manufacturer must establish and maintain instructions and procedures for performing service and verifying that the servicing meets specified requirements. Manufacturers have to analyze service reports with appropriate statistical methodology in accordance with their CAPA procedures. Service reports must be documented and include:

- The name of the device serviced

- Any device identification and control numbers used

- The date of service

- The individual(s) servicing the device

- The service performed

- The test and inspection data

If a manufacturer receives a service report that represents an event that must be reported to FDA, the report must be considered and dealt with as a complaint under QSR, as discussed above. The topics covered in Chapter 6, Post-Market Requirements, are particularly relevant to servicing issues and should be considered.

Section 2. Statistical Techniques

A manufacturer must have procedures for identifying valid statistical techniques required for establishing, controlling, and verifying the acceptance of process capability and product characteristics. Sampling plans must be written and based on valid statistical rationale and reviewed when changes are made, and these activities must be documented.

PART 13. QSIT INSPECTIONS

FDA conducts many types of medical device inspections of the regulated industry. Some examples include:

- QSIT inspections

- BIMO inspections

- Follow-up inspections to determine whether appropriate corrective actions were taken for deficiencies identified during a previous inspection

- "Directed" or "for cause" inspections when there is evidence that violations may have occurred at a regulated establishment

The two major inspections discussed in this book are QSIT inspections and BIMO inspections. The follow-up inspections and directed inspections are merely specialized versions of either the QSIT or BIMO inspections for a particular purpose. The BIMO inspections, or bioresearch monitoring inspections, are covered in Chapter 4, part 6, Bioresearch Monitoring, because the main focus of a BIMO inspection is the quality and integrity of a clinical trial.

On the other hand, a QSIT inspection is directed primarily at the quality and integrity of the manufacturing system. The QSIT inspection is the focus of this part of the book.

The term "QSIT" stands for *quality systems inspection technique*. FDA conducts many QSIT inspections under the QSR to assure compliance with these requirements. QSIT inspections are carried out by FDA investigators stationed in FDA's Regional and District Offices.

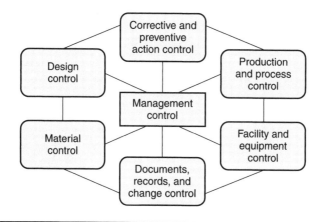

Figure 7.1 QSIT inspection subsystems.

FDA has guidance for agency staff on how to conduct a quality audit, what to look for, and actions to be taken. To accomplish such a daunting task, FDA has adopted a risk-based system in order to focus its inspectional resources in an efficient, yet effective, manner.

To accomplish this task, FDA has defined seven subsystems within the manufacturing process, as illustrated in Figure 7.1. FDA uses these subsystems for planning and carrying out its quality inspections. For a thorough description of the QSR inspectional system, see the FDA web page entitled "Inspections, Compliance, Enforcement, and Criminal Investigations" at:

http://www.fda.gov/ICECI/Inspections/InspectionGuides/ucm074883.htm#page7

Section 1. Conducting a QSIT Inspection

A QSIT inspection may be conducted at the establishments of manufacturers, distributors, suppliers, contract manufacturers, or any other places where regulated medical devices may be found. A BIMO inspection may be conducted at the site of the manufacturer, clinical site, IRB site, clinics, institutions, safety committees, and other related places involved in biomedical research with medical devices.

All of these inspection processes have certain steps in common even though the intent and object of an inspection may vary. Figure 7.2 represents the general inspection process that will be used by FDA, which is equally applicable to BIMO inspections.

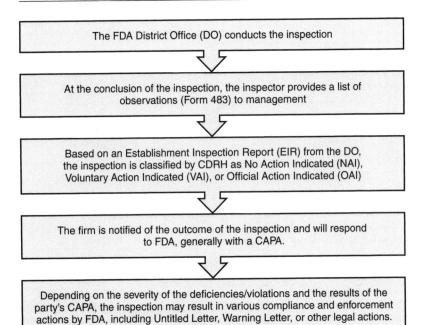

Figure 7.2   Medical device inspection process.

Types of QSIT Inspections

There are three types of QSIT inspections: level 1, level 2, and follow-up inspections. A level 1, or *abbreviated inspection,* covers the corrective and preventive action (CAPA) subsystem and either the design control or production and process control subsystem.

A level 2, or *baseline inspection,* covers four main subsystems. This inspection provides an overall evaluation of the firm's quality systems.

A compliance *follow-up inspection* is conducted to verify whether the corrections of previous violations are adequate, or to document continuing violations to support possible regulatory actions. It is conducted to follow up on information indicating serious problems at the firm, and it may include elements of a level 1 or level 2 inspection, as necessary.

Inspection Guides

FDA publishes the inspection guides that are used by FDA investigators for QSIT inspections on its website. The "Guide to Inspections of Medical Device Manufacturers" is located at:

http://www.fda.gov/ICECI/Inspections/InspectionGuides/
ucm074899.htm

There are also Inspection Technical Guides for areas such as quality systems and electromagnetic compatibility aspects of medical device quality systems, computers, electronic components, and others, which can be accessed from:

http://www.fda.gov/ICECI/Inspections/InspectionGuides/
InspectionTechnicalGuides/default.htm

Form 483 and the Establishment Inspection Report (EIR)

When the inspection is over, the FDA investigator will meet with the organization's management and discuss with them the findings of the inspection. Significant findings will be presented in writing on a Form 483. Management may respond in writing to the 483 on how they will deal with, or have dealt with, the findings. An adequate response from management to a 483 will contain the following elements:

* An assessment of the root cause of the problem

* An evaluation of the extent of the problem

* Any corrective actions to correct the problem

* The plan to institute any preventive actions to avoid recurrence

* Timelines for implementation

* Supporting documentation

The QSIT investigator will further prepare an Establishment Inspection Report (EIR), which will comprehensively set forth the details of the inspection and findings, including exhibits and documents.

Inspection Classification

The EIR will be sent to the CDRH for review and final classification. The inspection can result in the one of the following determinations by CDRH:

1. *No Action Indicated (NAI).* This determination is based on the fact that there were no objectionable conditions or practices.

2. *Voluntary Action Indicated (VAI).* This is based on the fact that there were objectionable conditions or practices but not so extensive that they meet the threshold to take or recommend administrative or regulatory action.

3. *Official Action Indicated (OAI)*. In this case, the inspection found serious objectionable conditions, and regulatory action is recommended and indicated.

Corrective and Preventive Actions

A manufacturer may have to undertake a CAPA to correct deficiencies or violations found during the QSIT inspection. Corrective actions are discussed above in Part 8, Corrective and Preventive Actions. The same CAPA principles and procedures are applicable whether the CAPA is undertaken to deal with in-process problems or to deal with problems arising after marketing a device. It is important to keep in mind that a CAPA may be used for deficiencies that have been found through the activities of the firm's internal quality system processes or discovered by FDA during an inspection.

Section 2. Examples of Violations Found During Inspections

There are many types of violations found during a QSIT inspection. They may be related to any of the QSR requirements discussed in this chapter and in Chapter 2, Medical Device Design. Examples of these violations can be found in the Warning Letters posted on the FDA website at:

http://www.fda.gov/ICECI/EnforcementActions/WarningLetters/default.htm#Recent

Below are four selections from these Warning Letters to medical device manufacturers issued by FDA in 2009. These examples illustrate the variety of violations found during a QSIT/QSR inspection.

Failure to Validate Packaging Changes and Other Changes

Letter to Dynamic Surgery, Inc., 10/13/09:

> Failure to perform and document revalidation activities when changes or process deviations occur in the manufacturing operations, as required by 21 CFR 820.75(c). For example, a packaging change was made for your cautery probes, LCP-14003 lot 090625, and there was no documentation to demonstrate that this new package did not affect the sterile integrity of the device. We also observed that you transferred packaging and manufacturing operations to two separate contract manufacturers. Your firm did not perform any revalidation activities to demonstrate that these significant changes compromised the integrity of the finished device.

Failures Related to Complaint Handling and MDR

Letter to Philips Healthcare, Inc., 10/9/09:

> Failure to establish and maintain adequate procedures for receiving, reviewing, and evaluating complaints by a formerly designated unit to ensure all complaints are processed in a uniform and timely manner, as required by 21 CFR 820.198(a)(1) . . . . For example: (b)(4), document number A-Q2920-00135, establishes that all complaints are to be handled in a timely manner with closure targeted for 90 days from the initiation date of the complaint. Observation 4a of the 483 report highlights several repairs and complaints regarding (b)(4) the external defibrillator using the (b)(4) prone to silver dendrites that were reported as early as August 27, 2007, but were not submitted as MDR to the FDA until January 21, 2009, beyond the 90-day target date for completion.

Failure to Evaluate Suppliers

Letter to Customed, Inc., 9/11/09:

> Failure to evaluate and select potential contractors on the basis of their ability to meet specified requirements as required by 21 CFR 820.50(a)(1). Specifically, your procedures to approve contract providers and external services failed to thoroughly assess the contract laboratory capability to perform the ETO residual test. The test methods used by the contract laboratory testing your products for ETO residuals refer to (b)(4). As discussed on item number 1 of this letter, composite sample-test of multi-devices systems is not contemplated within the referred standard. However, your firm has been accepting ETO residuals reported as a composite of samples from the devices within the kits. Moreover, no documentation was provided during the inspection to demonstrate that your firm assessed the capability of the laboratory contracted to conduct such analysis in conformance with the subject standards.

False and Misleading Labeling

Warning Letter issued to Baxter Healthcare Corp., 9/10/09:

> These inspections revealed that your (b)(4) is misbranded within the meaning of Section 502(a) of the Act [21 U.S.C. 352(a)], in that its labeling is false and misleading. Your package insert labeling for this device, which was approved under PMA (b)(4), states that (b)(4) are suspended in phosphate buffered saline with

(b)(4) United States Pharmacopeia (USP). However, the (b)(4) has been manufactured with (b)(4) since 1999.

Section 3. Third-Party Inspections

Inspections conducted by third parties and other regulators have been utilized by FDA in different circumstances. FDA utilizes these other inspectional findings because they provide a leveraging effect on FDA's limited inspectional resources.

Third-Party Inspection Program

The FDCA authorized a third-party inspection program under which FDA trains and accredits third parties, such as CROs and consulting firms, to perform inspections of eligible establishments that manufacture Class II or III devices. FDA refers to this third-party inspection program as the Accredited Persons (AP) Inspection Program. This is a voluntary program that firms may take advantage of for purposes of efficiency and timeliness. While all firms remain subject to inspection by FDA, eligible manufacturers have the option of requesting inspection by an AP. FDA has committed significant resources to creating the AP Inspection Program and continues to maintain it.

ISO Voluntary Audit Reports

FDA published in the *Federal Register (FR)* dated May 20, 2010, a draft guidance entitled, "Medical Device ISO 13485:2003 Voluntary Audit Report Submission Program." The *FR* notice may be reviewed at:

http://edocket.access.gpo.gov/2010/pdf/2010-12098.pdf

According to the preamble:

Under this draft guidance, device manufacturers whose establishment has been audited under one of the regulatory systems implemented by the Global Harmonization Task Force (GHTF) founding members using ISO 13485:2003 "Medical devices—Quality management systems—Requirements for regulatory purposes," may voluntarily submit the resulting audit report to FDA. If, based on that report, FDA determines there is minimal probability—in light of the relationship between the quality system deficiencies observed and the particular device and manufacturing processes involved—that the establishment will produce nonconforming and/or defective finished devices, then FDA intends to use the audit results as part of its risk assessment to determine whether that establishment can be removed from FDA's routine work plan for one year.

Under this proposal, if a qualified manufacturer has passed an inspection by a founding member of GHTF, which includes the auditing systems of the Canadian Medical Devices Conformity Assessment System, the European Union Notified Body accreditation system, the Therapeutic Goods Administration of Australia Inspectorate, and the Japanese Medical Device Ministry of Health, Labour and Welfare system, that manufacturer may submit the results to the FDA for consideration. Such reports will be used by CDRH and CBER in planning inspections for the upcoming year.

In this manner, the FDA may leverage audits performed by other GHTF regulators and accredited third parties in order to assist the agency in setting risk-based inspectional priorities.

PART 14. EXERCISES

1. Search the Internet for a definition of "quality" and explain why the definition you have chosen fits your concept of quality for a medical device.

2. Your career has been very successful, and you are one of the rising engineering stars of your company. The Quality Systems Oversight Committee is aware of problems that have arisen in the production of the contact lenses your company manufactures, and it fears they will not be able to pass an inspection by the FDA, which you expect in the near future. The committee has directed the various engineering teams to prepare new SOPs and protocols for use by the manufacturing department. Luckily, your team is the first one to be asked to prepare a manufacturing procedure, so you will be able to choose the SOP you wish to work on. Please select and prepare a manufacturing procedure that will be compliant with the requirements of the QSR. Also prepare an accompanying slide show for presentation to the Quality Systems Oversight Committee.

3. What are the actions management of a medical device manufacturer must take to fulfill its responsibilities under the QSR?

4. How should a manufacturer evaluate suppliers, contractors, and consultants?

5. If you were the manager of a manufacturing firm, what steps would you take to assure compliance with the QSR's requirements related to nonconforming product?

6. Under the QSR, manufacturers need procedures to identify existing and potential causes of nonconforming product or other quality problems and for implementing corrective and preventive actions (CAPA). What steps would you include in an SOP to assure that an acceptable corrective and preventive action plan is adopted and implemented?

7. Explain the labeling control requirements of the QSR.

8. What are the differences between the device master record (DMR) and the device history record (DHR)?

9. You are the sole proprietor of a consulting firm doing business as the Quality Systems Advisors, and you have been retained to advise a medical device manufacturer on a recently received Warning Letter (WL). From the FDA Warning Letter database, select a WL that includes violations of the QSR and prepare a corrective and preventive action plan for one of the QSR violations. In your CAPA, include the name of the firm, the date, and the name of the device. Present an analysis of the basis for the problem, and present your ideas for correcting and preventing the underlying problems. Include a draft SOP as well as a slide show for presentation to the company managers.

10. The medical device firm you work for has just undertaken a Class I recall of its automatic external defibrillator (AED). This device is used by emergency and medical personnel, or by others who have completed CPR AED training courses. It is intended to treat adults having a heart attack (cardiac arrest). The device analyzes an unconscious patient's heart rhythm and automatically delivers an electrical shock to the heart if needed to restore a normal heart rhythm. The device was recalled because it may experience:

    a. Low defibrillation energy delivery

    b. Unexpected device shutdown, and/or

    c. Inadequate filtering of electromagnetic noise

These failures could lead to a sudden stoppage of the device, may prevent defibrillation of a patient in cardiac arrest, and could lead to death.

The president of your company has asked you to explain how to deal with this recall.

11. You were just hired by the FDA District Office as an FDA investigator. For your first assignment, your branch chief informs you that you are going to be sent to a medical device facility to conduct a QSIT inspection. You are instructed to review the FDA inspection guide on the agency's website for guidance on conducting a QSIT inspection and to prepare an inspection plan on how you will conduct the inspection. Prepare your inspection plan for presentation to the branch chief for approval before embarking on your first inspection.

8

Compliance and Enforcement

O ne of FDA's major responsibilities for medical devices is to assure the regulated industry's compliance with applicable laws and regulations. Failure to meet the requirements of the FDCA and FDA regulations may result in FDA instituting an administrative, civil, or criminal action against the person or entity committing the violation or against the violative product. This chapter discusses topics that relate to FDA's compliance and enforcement activities and covers prohibited acts, mandatory recalls, general controls, compliance actions, and penalties.

PROHIBITED ACTS

FDA can undertake a compliance or enforcement action when it discovers that a regulated person is in violation of the FDCA or that a device is violative. The act sets forth various prohibited acts, the violation of which may serve as the basis for an administrative action or the institution of a civil or criminal proceeding.

The prohibited acts cover virtually all the requirements that are discussed throughout this book. They include the "general controls" discussed below in part 1, General Controls. Prohibited acts also cover failures to comply with "specific controls" such as those applicable to: Medical Device Design (Chapter 2), Nonclinical Testing (Chapter 3), Clinical Trials (Chapter 4), Marketing Applications (Chapter 5), Post-Approval Requirements (Chapter 6), and Quality Systems and GMPs (Chapter 7).

There are also a number of miscellaneous violations covered by prohibited acts, such as the falsification of a declaration of conformity to a standard. All of the prohibited acts that are enumerated in Section 301 of the FDCA are presented verbatim in Appendix B, Prohibited Acts, for those who wish to read them.

MANDATORY RECALLS

It should be noted in this chapter that FDA is heavily involved in the recall process because the recall process involves violative products already in commercial distribution where they may cause harm to patients or users. The agency will provide oversight over each recall, classify the recall, comment on the firm's strategy, review the firm's recall communications, witness a product's destruction or approve a reconditioning plan, and audit the general effectiveness of a recall.

The manufacturer has the primary responsibility to conduct a medical device recall. In fact, most recalls are voluntarily initiated and carried out by the manufacturer. Since the topic of voluntary recalls initiated by a manufacturer is discussed in detail as a post-approval requirement in Chapter 6, part 4, Medical Device Recalls, FDA's role in mandating a recall, although appropriate for discussion in this part, is included in Chapter 6 because it facilitates that discussion and avoids unnecessary repetition.

PART 1. GENERAL CONTROLS

The term "general controls" refers to a wide range of responsibilities and requirements that are applicable in general to manufacturers and others who are engaged in the medical device distribution system. General controls include requirements related to:

- Adulterated devices

- Misbranded devices

- Establishment registration

- Product listing

- Restrictions on the sale, distribution, or use of certain devices

- Premarket notification (510[k])

- Compliance with the Quality System Regulation (QSR)

- Record-keeping requirements

- Labeling requirements

- Medical device reporting (MDR)

- Notification of risks

- Recalls

- Repair, replacement, or refunds

Many of these topics have been covered in previous chapters. This chapter discusses some of these general controls that have not been covered elsewhere in the book.

Section 1. Adulterated Devices

The general and traditional definition of *adulterating* a product means an act of corrupting or debasing a product by incorporating an impure or spurious substance. The FDCA has an expanded definition of an adulterated device. Under this law, a device may be adulterated due to the defective nature of an intrinsic characteristic of the device itself. Other times, however, under the FDCA it may be due to the conditions surrounding the device even though there may be nothing intrinsically wrong with the device itself.

Intrinsic Qualities That Adulterate

The quality of the device may cause it to be adulterated if:

- It consists of any filthy, putrid, or decomposed substance.

- Its strength, purity, or quality does not comply with its label.

- It contains an unsafe color additive.

- It does not conform to applicable established performance standards.

External Conditions That Adulterate

Conditions external to the device will render it adulterated if:

- It was processed or held under unsanitary conditions.

- Its container is made of poisonous or deleterious materials.

- The facilities or controls for the manufacture, packaging, storage, process controls, record keeping, or installation do not meet applicable standards or conditions, for example, the QSR.

- It is offered for import to the United States, and the foreign manufacturer refused to be inspected by FDA.

- It is a banned device.

- It is an investigational device and it is not the subject of an approved investigational device exemption (IDE).

- It fails to comply with requirements related to its investigational status.

- It is a Class I or Class II device and it is not the subject of a cleared Premarket Notification (510[k]).

- It is a Class III device and it is not the subject of an approved:

  – Premarket Approval (PMA) application

  – A completed product development protocol (PDP), or

  – An approved humanitarian device exemption (HDE)

As explained elsewhere, a device does not have to be the subject of a cleared or approved application if it is a custom device, a device intended for research, a laboratory device, a device component, or supplies.

Section 2. Misbranded Device

In general terms, a *misbranded* product is one that contains false or misleading labeling. However, as with adulteration, the FDCA expands the conditions under which a medical device is deemed to be misbranded. A device may be considered to be misbranded due to the condition of its labeling or packaging, or it may be deemed to be misbranded because of conditions external to the actual label or packaging.

Packaging and Labeling Conditions That Cause Misbranding

The label or packaging will render a medical device misbranded if:

- Its labeling is false or misleading in any particular.

- The label does not include:

  – The name and address of the manufacturer, packer, or distributor

  – The quantity or measure of the contents

  – Adequate directions for use, with necessary patient protection warnings

  – The established name of the device

- It is dangerous to health if used as directed in the labeling

- Its packaging and labeling fail to meet any applicable color additive labeling or packaging requirements.

- It fails to meet the labeling requirements of an applicable standard.

- Its labeling does not contain the prescribed warning if the device is a restricted or prescription device, for example, "Caution: Federal law restricts this device to use by or on the order of a licensed practitioner."

Please note that there are exceptions for reasonable labeling variations, especially for small packages.

External Conditions That Cause Misbranding

A device may also be misbranded if:

- The advertisements for the device do not contain a brief statement of the intended uses of the device and relevant warnings, precautions, side effects, and contraindications.

- It was made in an establishment that did not meet certain registration requirements.

- The device is subject to post-market surveillance, and the manufacturer fails to comply with these requirements as ordered by FDA.

- There is a failure or refusal to comply with the MDR requirements.

- The manufacturer failed to comply with requirements of a PS order.

- The manufacturer or any distributor in the distribution chain failed to meet the tracking requirements.

Section 3. Registration and Listing

The owner or operator of a place of business (also called *establishments* or *facilities*) that is involved in the manufacture, preparation, propagation, compounding, assembly, or processing of a medical device intended for use in the United States is required to register annually with the FDA. The registration requirements apply to manufacturers, manufacturers of export-only devices, repackagers, relabelers, contract manufacturers who distribute the device, contract sterilizers who distribute the device, and kit assemblers.

Most establishments that are required to register with the FDA are also required to list the devices that are made there and the activities that are performed on those devices.

Registration and listing provide FDA with the location of medical device establishments and the devices manufactured at those establishments.

Knowing where devices are made increases the nation's ability to prepare for and respond to public health emergencies.

It should be noted that all FDA registration and listing must be done electronically unless FDA grants a waiver.

Section 4. Other General Controls

Some of the other general controls have already been discussed elsewhere along with the specific controls related to the topic under discussion. For example, premarket notification is itself a general control that involves extensive specific controls for the 510(k) program. Because these specific controls are so extensive and significant, both the general controls and the specific controls are covered together in Chapter 5, part 2, Premarket Notification (510[k]). Also, some general controls are included in the discussions in Chapter 6, Post-Market Requirements, and Chapter 7, Quality Systems and GMPs.

FDA provides additional advice on general controls on its website at:

http://www.fda.gov/MedicalDevices/DeviceRegulationand
Guidance/Overview/GeneralandSpecialControls/ucm055910.htm

PART 2. COMPLIANCE ACTIONS AND PENALTIES

There are many enforcement tools available to FDA when it finds a deficiency or violation of the FDCA or an FDA regulation. This part provides summary information about the compliance actions FDA can take and the types of penalties that may be applicable.

Section 1. Enforcement Discretion

FDA has finite resources with which to carry out its responsibilities under the FDCA. As discussed in Chapter 1, FDA allocates these resources among its premarket, post-market, compliance, and inspectional duties according to the needs of each area as dictated by conditions at that time. Similarly, within its compliance program, CDRH and its Office of Compliance have to make decisions on which violations it will pursue because there are not enough compliance resources available to take action against every infraction that is discovered. Under these circumstances, FDA must exercise what is referred to as "enforcement discretion."

In exercising this discretion, FDA will look at various factors before taking action. The following are some of the factors the agency will look at in determining whether a compliance action is indicated:

- The seriousness of the effect of the violation on patient safety

- The magnitude of the effect of the violation on the public health

- The effect of the infraction on undermining the integrity of the regulatory system

- Whether the act was intentional or inadvertent

- Previous violations by the same party

There are many examples of the agency exercising its enforcement discretion on the FDA website under the search term "enforcement discretion."

Section 2. Compliance Actions

FDA performs many tasks in carrying out its compliance responsibilities. For example, FDA inspects manufacturing facilities, investigates and evaluates complaints, oversees product recalls, orders notification, repair, replacement, or refund, and monitors the implementation of corrective and preventive actions.

FDA may conduct a variety of activities in support of its compliance responsibilities short of taking an action against a person or product. For example, the agency may hold "ad hocs," which are informal, internal committee meetings to conduct an in-depth examination of a particular issue of concern. It may conduct device inquiries to determine whether more-formal actions are required. FDA's laboratories (for medical devices it would be the CDRH Office of Science and Engineering Laboratories) may conduct research in support of compliance and evaluation activities. CDRH has a very active program of participation in the development of national and internal consensus standards for use by the industry and FDA.

When violative conduct is discovered, FDA has authority to pursue various administrative actions that are undertaken by the agency without resort to a court of law. Administrative actions may include the conduct of an administrative hearing. Administrative hearings are outlined in Chapter 1, part 6, FDA Administrative Actions

When the agency takes an administrative action, the regulated party may, in most cases after exhausting all administrative appeals and other administrative remedies, appeal to a court of law for review. Judicial review is outlined in Chapter 1, part 7, Judicial Review.

If the infractions are more serious and warrant the application of civil or criminal sanctions, the agency may resort to legal proceedings in a court of law.

Depending on the types of violations found, FDA may take any of the following administrative or legal actions. Which ones are sought depends on the seriousness of the problems, the risks they may pose to the safe use of the device, and the potential harm that may result from the use of the product. Each of the processes listed below are serious actions that have legal, business, and financial impacts for the party against whom the action is directed. There are varied and complex regulatory and legal requirements and restrictions attached to each action, which are beyond the scope of this book. The brief descriptions below are included because awareness of these potential actions may be instructive; however, when one of these actions is taken by FDA, legal representation is highly advisable.

Untitled and Warning Letters

Very often the first indication from FDA that there is a compliance problem is the issuance of an Untitled or Warning Letter to the affected party. These letters may be issued to persons or entities in the United States or to foreign importers. Warning Letters contain a listing of the actions or conditions that the agency considers violative. Failure on the part of the recipient of a Warning Letter to implement acceptable corrective actions may result in legal action by FDA. Sample excerpts from selected Warning Letters are included in Chapter 7, part 13, QSIT Inspections. The agency publishes all Warning Letters on its website at:

http://www.fda.gov/ICECI/EnforcementActions/WarningLetters/ default.htm

When FDA finds conditions that do not rise to the level of possible legal action, it may send an Untitled Letter to the party concerned, who is expected to undertake corrective actions. Failure to do so may invite further actions by the agency.

Mandatory Recalls

Mandatory recalls are discussed in Chapter 6, part 4, Medical Device Recalls

Notification, Repair, Replace, or Refund

This topic also has been covered in Chapter 6, part 5, Notification and Three R's.

Disqualification

Disqualification is a serious action by FDA that is not taken lightly or frequently by the agency. FDA may disqualify a person, such as a clinical investigator, a testing laboratory, a clinical site, or an IRB or its parent institution, if the FDA finds that person has been or is engaged in certain types of wrongdoing. The wrongdoing may involve:

- Repeated or deliberate violations of the agency's regulations

- The repeated or deliberate submission of false or misleading information to the sponsor or FDA in any required report, or

- Failure to take corrective actions that are or will be adequate to achieve compliance

A disqualification means that studies conducted by the disqualified person would not be acceptable in support of a submission to the agency. This could have a serious negative impact on any applications that contain study data from the disqualified person, and could affect any medical device firm using the services of the disqualified person. It may also prevent a disqualified person like a clinical investigator or testing lab from receiving an investigational device. A disqualified IRB would not be permitted to oversee clinical trials. Perhaps even more serious is the damage that would accrue to the reputation of the disqualified person once the scientific and business communities learn of the disqualification.

There are multiple steps that must be taken in arriving at a disqualification. Based on inspectional findings, FDA will issue a Form 483 of observations of deficiencies. Failure to correct the deficiencies will be followed by a Warning Letter. If the person fails to take appropriate corrective actions, and the agency determines that disqualification is the appropriate remedy, FDA will publish a public notice of the proposed disqualification action. After the disqualification process has been completed, the final decision by the agency will be published in the *Federal Register*. Along with disqualification, other regulatory, civil, or criminal actions may follow depending on the nature of the wrongdoing. To be reinstated, the disqualified person would have to provide assurances of future compliance.

Civil Money Penalties

FDA has the authority to administratively impose civil money penalties for violations of many device-related provisions of the FDCA. The penalties are assessed pursuant to a hearing before an administrative law judge. FDA can impose penalties up to $15,000 for each violation, totaling up to

$1,000,000 in each proceeding. Unpaid civil penalties can be collected by the Justice Department in an action in any appropriate federal district court.

Administrative Detention

If, during an inspection, FDA finds a device that it has "reason to believe" is adulterated or misbranded, the agency can order the device temporarily detained. This is an administrative action that temporarily prevents movement of a device while the agency seeks a seizure order from a court of law. The movement of a device in violation of the detention order, or the removal or alteration of a mark required by the order to identify the device as detained, is a prohibited act.

Seizure

Seizure of a medical device is conducted pursuant to a court order. An adulterated or misbranded device can be seized at any time without regard to whether the device is, or has been, in interstate commerce. The seizure may apply to a specific product, or to all models of a product, one or all lots, raw materials specific to the device, and in-process components. It generally does not apply to manufacturing equipment.

Embargo

FDA can refuse admission to the United States of a device if the device appears, among other things: (1) to be adulterated or misbranded, or (2) to be forbidden or restricted in sale in the country in which it was produced or from which it was exported. In such a case, the agency may place the device on import alert, preventing shipment of the product into the United States. At the appropriate time, a compliance follow-up inspection may be conducted. FDA typically reinspects a foreign manufacturer to confirm corrections before lifting an import alert. In some cases, FDA may first give the owner or consignee of the device a chance to recondition the device in order to bring it into compliance with the FDCA.

Injunction

An *injunction* is an order by a court requiring a person to do or to refrain from doing a specific act. The person may be an individual or a manufacturer or other enterprise. It may involve the manufacture or distribution of a device. The injunction may be a "preliminary" injunction that is effective during a 60-day period to allow the agency to file its complaint in court. A "permanent" injunction is a decree by the court after a hearing. A temporary restraining order (TRO) may be issued by the court prior to a full hearing if there is a risk of irreversible harm or the existence of a serious health hazard.

Criminal Prosecution

A prosecution is a criminal action directed against a firm or an individual. A conviction may result in fines or imprisonment or both. Fines can run up to $15,000 per violation and up to $1,000,000 per episode. In practice, fines of millions of dollars have been assessed against regulated firms for egregious and repeated infractions.

In addition to fines for criminal conduct, the FDCA provides for terms of imprisonment of one-year to 10-year periods, depending on the violation.

The U.S. criminal code, which is separate and apart from the FDCA, provides a wide range of penalties for violating its prohibitions, such as bribing a federal official or submitting a false statement of a material fact to a federal agency.

Consent Agreement

At any time before or during a compliance and enforcement action by FDA, the agency and the defendant may enter into a "consent decree," which is an agreement between the parties that contains details concerning the alleged violations, corrective actions that must be taken, future conduct, penalties that are applicable, and any other details necessary to resolve the issues between the parties. The consent agreement will be filed in court, and if the court agrees with the consent agreement, it will issue a decree embodying the consent agreement that will be enforceable through judicial actions.

Section 3. Regulatory Procedures Manual

FDA has a "Regulatory Procedures Manual" (RPM) available on the FDA website at:

> http://www.fda.gov/ora/compliance_ref/rpm/chapter2/ch2-2.
> html#SUB2-2-30

This manual describes the procedures that are available to the agency or that must be followed by FDA when instituting a compliance action. It also explains the rights of the person against whom an action is being taken.

PART 3. EXERCISES

1. Name the intrinsic qualities of a medical device that would render it adulterated.

2. Name conditions external to a medical device that would render it adulterated.

3. Under what conditions will the labeling or packaging render a medical device misbranded?

4. Explain the registration and listing requirements under general controls.

5. When FDA exercises its enforcement discretion, what are the factors the agency may look at in making its decision on whether to take action?

6. List the primary compliance actions available to FDA when it discovers violations of the FDCA and its regulations.

7. Search the FDA "Regulatory Procedures Manual" on the FDA website and select and discuss one of the compliance actions available to the agency. Indicate when such an action is appropriate, and its effect on the violator.

Appendix A
Website Links

N*ote:* This appendix contains a collection of all of the web pages cited throughout the text of *MDDR*. All of the websites in *MDDR* and this appendix were current when the text was prepared. However, FDA regularly updates its website, and some of the citations may change over time. It is, therefore, advisable to use appropriate search terms on the FDA website if the included citation does not yield the expected document.

Also, this appendix, with live hyperlinks, is being provided on a CD, which can be found inside the back cover. It may also be obtained via free download from the American Society for Quality's website at http://asq. org, or by e-mailing authors@asq.org. The CD or the downloaded appendix will allow a direct link to each of the listed websites, thus eliminating the need to type lengthy URLs in order to reach the desired web page.

Chapter 1—Background and Regulatory Environment

FDA Strategic Priorities web pages:

> http://www.fda.gov/AboutFDA/CentersOffices/CDRH/CDRH VisionandMission/ucm197647.htm

> http://www.fda.gov/AboutFDA/CentersOffices/CDRH/CDRH VisionandMission/ucm232531.htm

FDA Transparency Initiative task force home page:

> http://www.fda.gov/AboutFDA/WhatWeDo/FDATransparency TaskForce/default.htm

Division of Small Manufacturers, International and Consumer Assistance home page:

> http://www.fda.gov/medicaldevices/deviceregulationand
> guidance/ucm142656.htm

FDA Regulatory Procedures Manual:

> http://www.fda.gov/downloads/ICECI/ComplianceManuals/
> RegulatoryProceduresManual/UCM074340.pdf

Federal Food, Drug, and Cosmetic Act:

> http://www.fda.gov/opacom/laws/fdcact/fdctoc.htm

FDA guidance on Recognition and Use of Consensus Standards:

> http://www.fda.gov/downloads/MedicalDevices/Device
> RegulationandGuidance/GuidanceDocuments/ucm077295.pdf

FDA database of Recognized Standards:

> http://www.accessdata.fda.gov/scripts/cdrh/cfdocs/cfStandards/
> search.cfm

CDRH guidance documents:

> http://www.fda.gov/MedicalDevices/DeviceRegulationand
> Guidance/GuidanceDocuments/default.htm

FDA guidance documents:

> http://www.fda.gov/MedicalDevices/DeviceRegulationand
> Guidance/GuidanceDocuments/default.htm

Code of Federal Regulations Title 21 (FDA Regulations):

> http://www.accessdata.fda.gov/scripts/cdrh/cfdocs/cfcfr/
> cfrsearch.cfm

Connecticut Food, Drug, and Cosmetic Act:

> http://www.cga.ct.gov/2009/PUB/chap418.htm#Sec21a-91.htm

European Commission Consumer Affairs:

> http://ec.europa.eu/consumers/sectors/medical-devices/
> index_en.htm

LNE/G-MED's website (EU Notified Body):

> http://www.lne-gmed.com/en/services/ce-marking.asp

Global Harmonization Task Force website:

> http://www.ghtf.org/

HIPAA information from DHHS:

> http://www.hhs.gov/ocr/privacy/index.html

> http://www.hhs.gov/ocr/privacy/hipaa/understanding/
> coveredentities/research.html

IVD Regulatory Assistance:

> http://www.fda.gov/MedicalDevices/DeviceRegulationand
> Guidance/IVDRegulatoryAssistance/default.htm

Radiation-Emitting Products regulation:

> http://www.fda.gov/Radiation-EmittingProducts/default.htm

Device Classification:

> http://www.fda.gov/MedicalDevices/DeviceRegulationand
> Guidance/Overview/ClassifyYourDevice/default.htm

Product Code Classification Database:

> http://www.fda.gov/MedicalDevices/DeviceRegulationand
> Guidance/Overview/ClassifyYourDevice/ucm051637.htm

Medical Device Exemptions from 510(k) and GMP Requirements:

> http://www.accessdata.fda.gov/scripts/cdrh/cfdocs/cfpcd/315.cfm

Reserved Medical Devices:

> http://www.accessdata.fda.gov/scripts/cdrh/cfdocs/cfpcd/
> 3151.cfm

Chapter 2—Medical Device Design

Design Control Guidance for Medical Device Manufacturers:

> http://www.fda.gov/MedicalDevices/DeviceRegulationand
> Guidance/GuidanceDocuments/ucm070627.htm

Comparison of design standards and QSR requirements:

> http://elsmar.com/pdf_files/ISO-9001-2000-ISO-13485-2003-
> FDA-QSR-correspondence-matrix.pdf

Searchable device classification regulations:

> http://www.accessdata.fda.gov/scripts/cdrh/cfdocs/cfPCD/
> classification.cfm

Searchable cleared 510(k) database:

> http://www.accessdata.fda.gov/scripts/cdrh/cfdocs/cfpmn/
> pmn.cfm

List of Device Recalls:

> http://www.fda.gov/MedicalDevices/Safety/RecallsCorrections
> Removals/ListofRecalls/default.htm

Published Warning Letters:

> http://www.fda.gov/ICECI/EnforcementActions/WarningLetters/
> default.htm

FDA *Patient Safety News:*

> http://www.accessdata.fda.gov/scripts/cdrh/cfdocs/psn/index.cfm

Software validation guidance:

> http://www.fda.gov/downloads/MedicalDevices/Device
> RegulationandGuidance/GuidanceDocuments/UCM085371.pdf

FDA Luer locks letter:

> http://www.fda.gov/downloads/MedicalDevices/Resourcesfor
> You/Industry/UCM218631.pdf

Chapter 3—Nonclinical Testing

Finite Element Analysis: FDA guidance "Nonclinical Information for Femoral Stem Prostheses":

> http://www.fda.gov/MedicalDevices/DeviceRegulationand
> Guidance/GuidanceDocuments/ucm071275.htm

FDA guidance "Non-Clinical Engineering Tests and Recommended Labeling for Intravascular Stents and Associated Delivery Systems":

> http://www.fda.gov/MedicalDevices/DeviceRegulationand
> Guidance/GuidanceDocuments/ucm071863.htm

FDA guidance on biocompatibility testing:

http://www.fda.gov/MedicalDevices/DeviceRegulationand
Guidance/GuidanceDocuments/ucm080735.htm

Table 1 Initial Evaluation Tests for Consideration

Table 2 Supplementary Evaluation Tests for Consideration

FDA guidance "Container and Closure System Integrity Testing in Lieu of Sterility Testing as a Component of the Stability Protocol for Sterile Products":

http://www.fda.gov/RegulatoryInformation/Guidances/ucm
146074.htm

Chapter 4—Clinical Trials

"Protection of Human Subjects" (21 CFR Part 50):

http://www.accessdata.fda.gov/scripts/cdrh/cfdocs/cfcfr/
CFRSearch.cfm?CFRPart=50&showFR=1

"Financial Disclosure by Clinical Investigators" (21 CFR Part 54):

http://www.accessdata.fda.gov/scripts/cdrh/cfdocs/cfcfr/
CFRSearch.cfm?CFRPart=54&showFR=1

"Institutional Review Boards" (21 CFR Part 56):

http://www.accessdata.fda.gov/scripts/cdrh/cfdocs/cfcfr/
CFRSearch.cfm?CFRPart=56&showFR=1

"Investigational Device Exemptions" (21 CFR Part 812):

http://www.accessdata.fda.gov/scripts/cdrh/cfdocs/cfcfr/
CFRSearch.cfm?CFRPart=812&showFR=1

Quality System Regulation—Design Controls (21 CFR Part 820 Subpart C):

http://www.accessdata.fda.gov/scripts/cdrh/cfdocs/cfcfr/
CFRSearch.cfm?CFRPart=820&showFR=1

"Electronic Records; Electronic Signatures" (21 CFR Part 11):

http://www.accessdata.fda.gov/scripts/cdrh/cfdocs/cfCFR/
CFRSearch.cfm?CFRPart=11

NIH Fact Sheet "Registration at ClinicalTrials.gov: As Required by Public Law 110-85, Title VIII":

> http://prsinfo.clinicaltrials.gov/s801-fact-sheet.pdf

CODEX compilation of international standards for clinical research:

> http://www.codex.vr.se/en/forskningmedicin.shtml

NIH guidance "Ethics in Clinical Research":

> http://clinicalresearch.nih.gov/ethics_guides.html

NIH Slides "What Makes Clinical Research Ethical?":

> http://www.bioethics.nih.gov/slides/10-29-03-Emmanuel.pdf

NIH proposed regulations on financial interests:

> http://www.gpo.gov/fdsys/pkg/FR-2010-05-21/pdf/2010-11885.pdf

FDA guidance "Informed Consent for In Vitro Diagnostic Device Studies Using Leftover Human Specimens That Are Not Individually Identifiable":

> http://www.fda.gov/MedicalDevices/DeviceRegulationand
> Guidance/GuidanceDocuments/ucm078384.htm

FDA guidance "Establishment and Operation of Clinical Trial Data Monitoring Committees":

> http://www.fda.gov/downloads/RegulatoryInformation/
> Guidances/ucm127073.pdf

Bioresearch Monitoring program:

> http://www.fda.gov/ora/compliance_ref/bimo/

Clinical trials protocol registration system:

> http://www.clinicaltrials.gov

NIH fact sheet "Registration at ClinicalTrials.gov: As Required by Public Law 110-85, Title VIII":

> http://prsinfo.clinicaltrials.gov/s801-fact-sheet.pdf

Chapter 5—Marketing Applications

"Summary FDA Review Memos for 180-Day Design Changes":

http://www.fda.gov/AboutFDA/CentersOffices/CDRH/
CDRHTransparency/ucm206289.htm

FDA guidance "Human Factors Principles for Medical Device Labeling":

http://www.fda.gov/downloads/MedicalDevices/Device
RegulationandGuidance/GuidanceDocuments/UCM095300.pdf

"Sample Panel Pack Materials for Upcoming Panel Meeting":

http://www.fda.gov/AdvisoryCommittees/CommitteesMeeting
Materials/MedicalDevices/MedicalDevicesAdvisoryCommittee/
CirculatorySystemDevicesPanel/ucm240575.htm

"Application Integrity Policy":

http://www.fda.gov/downloads/ICECI/EnforcementActions/
ApplicationIntegrityPolicy/UCM072631.pdf

"Electronic Copies for Premarket Submissions":

http://www.fda.gov/MedicalDevices/DeviceRegulationand
Guidance/HowtoMarketYourDevice/PremarketSubmissions/
ucm134508.htm

FDA guidance "Medical Device User Fee and Modernization Act (MDUFMA)":

http://www.fda.gov/MedicalDevices/DeviceRegulationand
Guidance/Overview/MedicalDeviceUserFeeandModernization
ActMDUFMA/default.htm

FDA guidance "User Fees and Refunds for Premarket Notification Submissions (510[k]s)":

http://www.fda.gov/MedicalDevices/DeviceRegulationand
Guidance/GuidanceDocuments/ucm089753.htm

CDRH Premarket Review Submission Cover Sheet:

http://www.fda.gov/downloads/AboutFDA/ReportsManuals
Forms/Forms/UCM080872.pdf

Premarket Notification 510(k) home page:

> http://www.fda.gov/MedicalDevices/DeviceRegulationand
> Guidance/HowtoMarketYourDevice/PremarketSubmissions/
> PremarketNotification510k/default.htm

"The New 510(k) Paradigm":

> http://www.fda.gov/MedicalDevices/DeviceRegulationand
> Guidance/GuidanceDocuments/ucm080187.htm

"510(k) Submission Process":

> http://www.fda.gov/MedicalDevices/DeviceRegulationand
> Guidance/HowtoMarketYourDevice/PremarketSubmissions/
> PremarketNotification510k/ucm070201.htm

"510(k) Review Template":

> http://www.fda.gov/MedicalDevices/DeviceRegulationand
> Guidance/HowtoMarketYourDevice/PremarketSubmissions/
> PremarketNotification510k/ucm071420.htm

"510(k) 'Substantial Equivalence' Decision Making Process" flowchart:

> http://www.fda.gov/MedicalDevices/DeviceRegulationand
> Guidance/HowtoMarketYourDevice/PremarketSubmissions/
> PremarketNotification510k/ucm134783.htm

Releasable 510(k) database:

> http://www.fda.gov/MedicalDevices/ProductsandMedical
> Procedures/DeviceApprovalsandClearances/510kClearances/
> ucm089319.htm

510(k) Premarket Notification database search screen:

> http://www.accessdata.fda.gov/scripts/cdrh/cfdocs/cfPMN/
> pmn.cfm

"Screening Checklist for Traditional/Abbreviated Premarket Notification (510[k]) Submissions":

> http://www.fda.gov/MedicalDevices/DeviceRegulationand
> Guidance/HowtoMarketYourDevice/PremarketSubmissions/
> PremarketNotification510k/ucm071360.htm

Steps in the 510(k) submission process:

> http://www.fda.gov/MedicalDevices/DeviceRegulationand
> Guidance/HowtoMarketYourDevice/PremarketSubmissions/
> PremarketNotification510k/ucm070201.htm

"510(k) 'Substantial Equivalence' Decision Making Process" flowchart:

> http://www.fda.gov/MedicalDevices/DeviceRegulationand
> Guidance/HowtoMarketYourDevice/PremarketSubmissions/
> PremarketNotification510k/ucm134783.htm

Listing of FDA-accredited third-party reviewers:

> http://www.accessdata.fda.gov/scripts/cdrh/cfdocs/cfthirdparty/
> accredit.cfm

Listing of devices eligible for third-party review:

> http://www.accessdata.fda.gov/scripts/cdrh/cfdocs/cfThirdParty/
> current.cfm

510(k) confidentiality provisions [NOTE: In the search box type "807.95" for the "Confidentiality of Information" for 510(k)s]:

> http://www.accessdata.fda.gov/scripts/cdrh/cfdocs/cfcfr/
> CFRSearch.cfm

"CDRH Preliminary Internal Evaluations" home page:

> http://www.fda.gov/AboutFDA/CentersOffices/CDRH/
> CDRHReports/ucm220272.htm

"Premarket Approval (PMA)" home page:

> http://www.fda.gov/MedicalDevices/DeviceRegulationand
> Guidance/HowtoMarketYourDevice/PremarketSubmissions/
> PremarketApprovalPMA/default.htm

Sample PMA cover sheet:

> http://www.fda.gov/ohrms/dockets/ac/02/briefing/3910b1_08_
> summary%20data.doc

Sample SSED:

> http://www.fda.gov/ohrms/dockets/dockets/04m0471/04m-0471-
> cr00001-02-SSED-vol42.pdf

Guidance on the preparation and content of a PMA, including an SSED:

> http://www.fda.gov/MedicalDevices/DeviceRegulationand
> Guidance/HowtoMarketYourDevice/PremarketSubmissions/
> PremarketApprovalPMA/ucm050289.htm

Guidance on day-100 PMA meetings:

> http://www.fda.gov/MedicalDevices/DeviceRegulationand
> Guidance/GuidanceDocuments/ucm080190.htm

Searchable list of annual PMA approvals:

> http://www.fda.gov/MedicalDevices/ProductsandMedical
> Procedures/DeviceApprovalsandClearances/PMAApprovals/
> ucm096300.htm

"PMA Post-Approval Requirements":

> http://www.fda.gov/MedicalDevices/DeviceRegulationand
> Guidance/HowtoMarketYourDevice/PremarketSubmissions/
> PremarketApprovalPMA/ucm050422.htm

"Post-Approval Studies" database:

> http://www.accessdata.fda.gov/scripts/cdrh/cfdocs/cfPMA/pma_
> pas.cfm

FDA guidance "Modifications to Devices Subject to Premarket Approval (PMA)—The PMA Supplement Decision-Making Process," including "Figure 1. Recommended Steps to Decide the Regulatory Path for a Modified PMA Device.":

> http://www.fda.gov/MedicalDevices/DeviceRegulationand
> Guidance/GuidanceDocuments/ucm089274.htm

FDA guidance "Real-Time Premarket Approval Application (PMA) Supplements":

> http://www.fda.gov/MedicalDevices/DeviceRegulationand
> Guidance/GuidanceDocuments/ucm089602.htm

Guidance on 30-day notices and 135-day PMA supplements:

> http://www.fda.gov/MedicalDevices/DeviceRegulationand
> Guidance/GuidanceDocuments/ucm080192.htm

FDA "Guidance for HDE Holders, Institutional Review Boards (IRBs), Clinical Investigators, and FDA Staff—Humanitarian Device Exemption (HDE) Regulation: Questions and Answers":

> http://www.fda.gov/MedicalDevices/DeviceRegulationand Guidance/GuidanceDocuments/ucm110194.htm

FDA guidance "Importing and Exporting Devices":

> http://www.fda.gov/MedicalDevices/DeviceRegulationand Guidance/ImportingandExportingDevices/default.htm

Medical device export flowchart:

> http://www.fda.gov/MedicalDevices/DeviceRegulationand Guidance/ImportingandExportingDevices/ucm050521. htm#flowchart

Chapter 6—Post-Market Requirements

FDA guidance "Medical Device Reporting for Manufacturers":

> http://www.fda.gov/MedicalDevices/DeviceRegulationand Guidance/GuidanceDocuments/ucm094529.htm#elect

MDR MedWatch forms:

> http://www.fda.gov/Safety/MedWatch/HowToReport/ DownloadForms/default.htm

Searchable database of Medical Device Reports:

> http://www.fda.gov/MedicalDevices/Safety/ReportaProblem/ ucm124073.htm

FDA guidance "Postmarket Surveillance under Section 522 of the Federal Food, Drug, and Cosmetic Act":

> http://www.fda.gov/MedicalDevices/DeviceRegulationand Guidance/GuidanceDocuments/ucm072517.htm

Listing of Section 522 post-market surveillance studies:

> http://www.accessdata.fda.gov/scripts/cdrh/cfdocs/cfPMA/ pss.cfm

FDA "Guidance for Industry: Product Recalls, Including Removals and Corrections":

> http://www.fda.gov/Safety/Recalls/IndustryGuidance/ucm
> 129259.htm

FDA lists of device recalls:

> http://www.fda.gov/MedicalDevices/Safety/RecallsCorrections
> Removals/ListofRecalls/default.htm

> http://www.fda.gov/Safety/Recalls/default.htm

"MedWatch Safety Alerts for Human Medical Products":

> http://www.fda.gov/Safety/MedWatch/SafetyInformation/
> SafetyAlertsforHumanMedicalProducts/default.htm

"Health Hazard Evaluation Form":

> http://www.fda.gov/MedicalDevices/DeviceRegulationand
> Guidance/IVDRegulatoryAssistance/ucm126206.htm

Searchable recall database:

> http://www.accessdata.fda.gov/scripts/cdrh/cfdocs/cfRES/
> res.cfm

Chapter 7—Quality Systems and GMPs

Article on quality:

> http://en.wikipedia.org/wiki/Quality_(business)

FDA Warning Letters:

> http://www.fda.gov/ICECI/EnforcementActions/WarningLetters/
> default.htm#Recent

"Inspections, Compliance, Enforcement, and Criminal Investigations":

> http://www.fda.gov/ICECI/Inspections/InspectionGuides/
> ucm074883.htm#page7

Guide to inspections of medical device manufacturers:

> http://www.fda.gov/ICECI/Inspections/InspectionGuides/
> ucm074899.htm

"Inspection Technical Guides":

http://www.fda.gov/ICECI/Inspections/InspectionGuides/
InspectionTechnicalGuides/default.htm

Searchable Warning Letters database:

http://www.fda.gov/ICECI/EnforcementActions/Warning
Letters/default.htm#Recent

FDA "Draft" guidance "Medical Device ISO 13485:2003 Voluntary Audit
Report Submission Program":

http://edocket.access.gpo.gov/2010/pdf/2010-12098.pdf

Chapter 8—Compliance and Enforcement

FDA advice "General Controls for Medical Devices":

http://www.fda.gov/MedicalDevices/DeviceRegulationand
Guidance/Overview/GeneralandSpecialControls/ucm055910.htm

Searchable Warning Letters database:

http://www.fda.gov/ICECI/EnforcementActions/WarningLetters/
default.htm#Recent

"Regulatory Procedures Manual":

http://www.fda.gov/ora/compliance_ref/rpm/chapter2/ch2-2.
html#SUB2-2-30

Appendix B
Prohibited Acts

N*ote:* This appendix is a verbatim reproduction of Section 301 of the Federal Food, Drug, and Cosmetic Act. It covers all products regulated by FDA and applies specifically to medical devices as stated in the text. It can be found at:

SEC. 301. [21 USC §331] Prohibited acts

SEC. 301. [21 USC §331] PROHIBITED ACTS

Note: revisions were posted to this section in February 2008.

The following acts and the causing thereof are hereby prohibited:[1]

(a) The introduction or delivery for introduction into interstate commerce of any food, drug, device, or cosmetic that is adulterated or misbranded.

(b) The adulteration or misbranding of any food, drug, device, or cosmetic in interstate commerce.

(c) The receipt in interstate commerce of any food, drug, device, or cosmetic that is adulterated or misbranded, and the delivery or proffered delivery thereof for pay or otherwise.

(d) The introduction or delivery for introduction into interstate commerce of any article in violation of section 404, 505 or 564.

(e) The refusal to permit access to or copying of any record as required by section 412, 414, 416, 417(g), 504, 564, 703, 704(a), 760, or 761; or the failure to establish or maintain any record, or make any report, required under section 412, 414(b), 416, 417, 504, 505(i) or (k), 512(a)(4)(C), 512 (j), (l) or (m), 572(i),[2] 515(f), 519, 564, 760, or 761 or the refusal to permit access to or verification or copying of any such required record.

(f) The refusal to permit entry or inspection as authorized by section 704.

(g) The manufacture, within any Territory of any food, drug, device, or cosmetic that is adulterated or misbranded.

(h) The giving of a guaranty or undertaking referred to in section 303(c)(2), which guaranty or undertaking is false, except by a person who relied upon a guaranty or undertaking to the same effect signed by, containing the name and address of, the person residing in the United States from whom he received in good faith the food, drug, device, or cosmetic; or the giving of a guaranty or undertaking referred to in section 303(c)(3), which guaranty or undertaking is false.

(i) (1) Forging, counterfeiting, simulating, or falsely representing, or without proper authority using any mark, stamp, tag, label, or other identification device authorized or required by regulations promulgated under the provisions of section 404 or 721.

(2) Making, selling, disposing of, or keeping in possession, control, or custody, or concealing any punch, die, plate, stone, or other thing designed to print, imprint, or reproduce the trademark, trade name, or other identifying mark, imprint, or device of another or any likeness of any of the foregoing upon any drug or container or labeling thereof so as to render such drug a counterfeit drug.

(3) The doing of any act which causes a drug to be a counterfeit drug, or the sale or dispensing, or the holding for sale or dispensing, of a counterfeit drug.

(j) The using by any person to his own advantage or revealing, other than to the Secretary or officers or employees of the Department, or to the courts when relevant in any judicial proceeding under this Act, any information acquired under authority of section 404, 409, 412, 414, 505, 510, 512, 513, 514, 515, 516, 518, 519, 520, 571, 572, 573,[3] 704, 708, or 721 concerning any method or process which as a trade secret is entitled to protection; or the violating of section 408(i)(2) or any regulation issued under that section.[4] This paragraph does not authorize the withholding of information from either House of Congress or from, to the extent of matter within its jurisdiction, any committee or subcommittee of such committee or any joint committee of Congress or any subcommittee of such joint committee.

(k) The alteration, mutilation, destruction, obliteration, or removal of the whole or any part of the labeling of, or the doing of any other act with respect to, a food, drug, device, or cosmetic, if such act is done while such article is held for sale (whether or not the first sale) after shipment in interstate commerce and results in such article being adulterated or misbranded.

(l) [Deleted][5]

(m) The sale or offering for sale of colored oleomargarine or colored margarine, or the possession or serving of colored oleomargarine or colored margarine in violation of sections 407(b) or 407(c).

(n) The using, in labeling, advertising, or other sales promotion of any reference to any report or analysis furnished in compliance with section 704.

(o) In the case of a prescription drug distributed or offered for sale in interstate commerce, the failure of the manufacturer, packer, or distributor thereof to maintain for transmittal, or to transmit, to any practitioner licensed by applicable State law to administer such drug who makes written request for information as to such drug, true and correct copies of all printed matter which is required to be included in any package in which that drug is distributed or sold, or such other printed matter as is approved by the Secretary. Nothing in this paragraph shall be construed to exempt any person from any labeling requirement imposed by or under other provisions of this Act.

(p) The failure to register in accordance with section 510, the failure to provide any information required by section 510(j) or 510(k), 21 USC § 360(j) or (k)] or the failure to provide a notice required by section 510(j)(2).

(q)(1) The failure or refusal to (A) comply with any requirement prescribed under section 518 or 520(g), (B) furnish any notification or other material or information required by or under section 519 or 520(g), or (C) comply with a requirement under section 522.

(2) With respect to any device, the submission of any report that is required by or under this Act that is false or misleading in any material respect.

(r) The movement of a device in violation of an order under section 304(g) or the removal or alteration of any mark or label required by the order to identify the device as detained.

(s) The failure to provide the notice required by section 412(c) or 412(e), the failure to make the reports required by section 412(f)(1)(B), the failure to retain the records required by section 412(b)(4), or the failure to meet the requirements prescribed under section 412(f)(3).

(t) The importation of a drug in violation of section 801(d)(1), the sale, purchase, or trade of a drug or drug sample or the offer to sell, purchase, or trade a drug or drug sample in violation of section 503(c), the sale, purchase, or trade of a coupon, the offer to sell, purchase, or trade such a coupon, or the counterfeiting of such a coupon in violation of section 503(c)(2), the distribution of a drug sample in violation of section 503(d) or the failure to otherwise comply with the requirements of section 503(d), or the distribution of drugs in violation of section 503(e) or the failure to otherwise comply with the requirements of section 503(e).

(u) The failure to comply with any requirements of the provisions of, or any regulations or orders of the Secretary, under section 512(a)(4)(A), 512(a)(4)(D), or 512(a)(5).

(v) The introduction or delivery for introduction into interstate commerce of a dietary supplement that is unsafe under section 413.

(w) The making of a knowingly false statement in any statement, certificate of analysis, record, or report required or requested under section 801(d)(3); the failure to submit a certificate of analysis as required under such section; the failure to maintain records or to submit records or reports as required by such section; the release into interstate commerce of any article or portion thereof imported into the United States under such section or any finished product made from such article or portion, except for export in accordance with section 801(e) or 802, or with section 351(h) of the Public Health Service Act [42 USC § 262(h)]; or the failure to so export or to destroy such an article or portions thereof, or such a finished product.

(x) The falsification of a declaration of conformity submitted under section 514(c) or the failure or refusal to provide data or information requested by the Secretary under paragraph (3) of such section.

(y) In the case of a drug, device, or food—

(1) the submission of a report or recommendation by a person accredited under section 523 that is false or misleading in any material respect;

(2) the disclosure by a person accredited under section 523 of confidential commercial information or any trade secret without the express written consent of the person who submitted such information or secret to such person; or

(3) the receipt by a person accredited under section 523 of a bribe in any form or the doing of any corrupt act by such person associated with a responsibility delegated to such person under this Act.

(z) [Terminated][6]

(aa) The importation of a prescription drug in violation of section 804, the falsification of any record required to be maintained or provided to the Secretary under section, or any other violation of regulations under such section.

(bb) The transfer of an article of food in violation of an order under section 304(h), or the removal or alteration of any mark or label required by the order to identify the article as detained.

(cc) The importing or offering for import into the United States of an article of food by, with the assistance of, or at the direction of, a person debarred under section 306(b)(3).

(dd) The failure to register in accordance with section 415.

(ee) The importing or offering for import into the United States of an article of food in violation of the requirements under section 801(m).

(ff) The importing or offering for import into the United States of a drug or device with respect to which there is a failure to comply with a request of the Secretary to submit to the Secretary a statement under section 801(o).

(gg) The knowing failure to comply with paragraph (7)(E) of section 704(g); the knowing inclusion by a person accredited under paragraph (2) of such section of false information in an inspection report under paragraph (7)(A) of such section; or the knowing failure of such a person to include material facts in such a report.

(hh) The failure by a shipper, carrier by motor vehicle or rail vehicle, receiver, or any other person engaged in the transportation of food to comply with the sanitary transportation practices prescribed by the Secretary under section 416.

(ii) The falsification of a report of a serious adverse event submitted to a responsible person (as defined under section 760 or 761) or the falsification of a serious adverse event report (as defined under section 760 or 761) submitted to the Secretary.

(jj) (1) The failure to submit the certification required by section 402(j)(5)(B) of the Public Health Service Act [42 USC § 282(j)(5)(B)], or knowingly submitting a false certification under such section.

(2) The failure to submit clinical trial information required under subsection (j) of section 402 of the Public Health Service Act [42 USC § 282].

(3) The submission of clinical trial information under subsection (j) of section 402 of the Public Health Service Act [42 USC § 282] that is false or misleading in any particular under paragraph (5)(D) of such subsection (j).

(kk) *[Note: This subsection takes effect 180 days after enactment of Act Sept. 27, 2007, P.L. 110-85, as provided by § 909(a) of such Act, which appears as a note to this section.]* The dissemination of a television advertisement without complying with section 503B [21 USC § 353b].

(ll) The introduction or delivery for introduction into interstate commerce of any food to which has been added a drug approved under section 505 [21 USC § 355], a biological product licensed under section 351 of the Public Health Service Act [42 USC § 262], or a drug or a biological product for which substantial clinical investigations have been instituted and for which the existence of such investigations has been made public, unless—

(1) such drug or such biological product was marketed in food before any approval of the drug under section 505 [21 USC § 355], before licensure of the biological product under such section 351 [42 USC § 262], and

before any substantial clinical investigations involving the drug or the biological product have been instituted;

(2) the Secretary, in the Secretary's discretion, has issued a regulation, after notice and comment, approving the use of such drug or such biological product in the food;

(3) the use of the drug or the biological product in the food is to enhance the safety of the food to which the drug or the biological product is added or applied and not to have independent biological or therapeutic effects on humans, and the use is in conformity with—

(A) a regulation issued under section 409 [21 USC § 348] prescribing conditions of safe use in food;

(B) a regulation listing or affirming conditions under which the use of the drug or the biological product in food is generally recognized as safe;

(C) the conditions of use identified in a notification to the Secretary of a claim of exemption from the premarket approval requirements for food additives based on the notifier's determination that the use of the drug or the biological product in food is generally recognized as safe, provided that the Secretary has not questioned the general recognition of safety determination in a letter to the notifier;

(D) a food contact substance notification that is effective under section 409(h) [21 USC § 348(h)]; or

(E) such drug or biological product had been marketed for smoking cessation prior to the date of the enactment of the Food and Drug Administration Amendments Act of 2007 [enacted Sept. 27, 2007]; or

(4) the drug is a new animal drug whose use is not unsafe under section 512 [21 USC § 360b].

(mm) The failure to submit a report or provide a notification required under section 417(d) [21 USC § 350f(d)].

(nn) The falsification of a report or notification required under section 417(d) [21 USC § 350f(d)].

FOOTNOTES

1. See *footnote for section 403(h)(3)* regarding the stylistic use of a list consisting of "(a)," "(b)," etc.

2. The period is so in law. See section 102(b)(5)(C) of Public Law 108-282

3. The period is so in law. See section 102f(b)(5)(D) of Public Law 108-282.

4. So in law. See the amendment made by section 403 of Public Law 104–170 (110 Stat. 1514).

5. Paragraph (l) was struck by section 421 of Public Law 105–115 (111 Stat. 2380).

6. Paragraph (z) was added by subsection (b) of section 401(b) of Public Law 105–115 (111 Stat. 2364). Subsection (e) of such section provides as follows:

   (e) SUNSET.—The amendments made by this section cease to be effective September 30, 2006, or 7 years after the date on which the Secretary promulgates the regulations described in subsection (c), whichever is later.

Index

Belong to the Quality Community!

Established in 1946, ASQ is a global community of quality experts in all fields and industries. ASQ is dedicated to the promotion and advancement of quality tools, principles, and practices in the workplace and in the community.

The Society also serves as an advocate for quality. Its members have informed and advised the U.S. Congress, government agencies, state legislatures, and other groups and individuals worldwide on quality-related topics.

Vision

By making quality a global priority, an organizational imperative, and a personal ethic, ASQ becomes the community of choice for everyone who seeks quality technology, concepts, or tools to improve themselves and their world.

ASQ is...

- More than 90,000 individuals and 700 companies in more than 100 countries
- The world's largest organization dedicated to promoting quality
- A community of professionals striving to bring quality to their work and their lives
- The administrator of the Malcolm Baldrige National Quality Award
- A supporter of quality in all sectors including manufacturing, service, healthcare, government, and education
- YOU

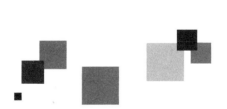

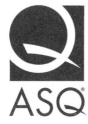

Visit www.asq.org for more information.

ASQ Membership

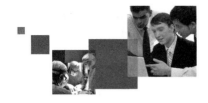

Research shows that people who join associations experience increased job satisfaction, earn more, and are generally happier*. ASQ membership can help you achieve this while providing the tools you need to be successful in your industry and to distinguish yourself from your competition. So why wouldn't you want to be a part of ASQ?

Networking

Have the opportunity to meet, communicate, and collaborate with your peers within the quality community through conferences and local ASQ section meetings, ASQ forums or divisions, ASQ Communities of Quality discussion boards, and more.

Professional Development

Access a wide variety of professional development tools such as books, training, and certifications at a discounted price. Also, ASQ certifications and the ASQ Career Center help enhance your quality knowledge and take your career to the next level.

Solutions

Find answers to all your quality problems, big and small, with ASQ's Knowledge Center, mentoring program, various e-newsletters, *Quality Progress* magazine, and industry-specific products.

Access to Information

Learn classic and current quality principles and theories in ASQ's Quality Information Center (QIC), *ASQ Weekly* e-newsletter, and product offerings.

Advocacy Programs

ASQ helps create a better community, government, and world through initiatives that include social responsibility, Washington advocacy, and Community Good Works.

Visit www.asq.org/membership for more information on ASQ membership.

*2008, The William E. Smith Institute for Association Research

ASQ Certification

ASQ certification is formal recognition by ASQ that an individual has demonstrated a proficiency within, and comprehension of, a specified body of knowledge at a point in time. Nearly 150,000 certifications have been issued. ASQ has members in more than 100 countries, in all industries, and in all cultures. ASQ certification is internationally accepted and recognized.

Benefits to the Individual

- New skills gained and proficiency upgraded
- Investment in your career
- Mark of technical excellence
- Assurance that you are current with emerging technologies
- Discriminator in the marketplace
- Certified professionals earn more than their uncertified counterparts
- Certification is endorsed by more than 125 companies

Benefits to the Organization

- Investment in the company's future
- Certified individuals can perfect and share new techniques in the workplace
- Certified staff are knowledgeable and able to assure product and service quality

Quality is a global concept. It spans borders, cultures, and languages. No matter what country your customers live in or what language they speak, they demand quality products and services. You and your organization also benefit from quality tools and practices. Acquire the knowledge to position yourself and your organization ahead of your competition.

Certifications Include
- Biomedical Auditor – CBA
- Calibration Technician – CCT
- HACCP Auditor – CHA
- Pharmaceutical GMP Professional – CPGP
- Quality Inspector – CQI
- Quality Auditor – CQA
- Quality Engineer – CQE
- Quality Improvement Associate – CQIA
- Quality Technician – CQT
- Quality Process Analyst – CQPA
- Reliability Engineer – CRE
- Six Sigma Black Belt – CSSBB
- Six Sigma Green Belt – CSSGB
- Software Quality Engineer – CSQE
- Manager of Quality/Organizational Excellence – CMQ/OE

Visit www.asq.org/certification to apply today!

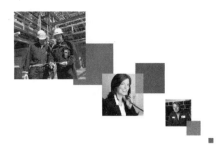

ASQ Training

Classroom-based Training

ASQ offers training in a traditional classroom setting on a variety of topics. Our instructors are quality experts and lead courses that range from one day to four weeks, in several different cities. Classroom-based training is designed to improve quality and your organization's bottom line. Benefit from quality experts; from comprehensive, cutting-edge information; and from peers eager to share their experiences.

Web-based Training

Virtual Courses

ASQ's virtual courses provide the same expert instructors, course materials, interaction with other students, and ability to earn CEUs and RUs as our classroom-based training, without the hassle and expenses of travel. Learn in the comfort of your own home or workplace. All you need is a computer with Internet access and a telephone.

Self-paced Online Programs

These online programs allow you to work at your own pace while obtaining the quality knowledge you need. Access them whenever it is convenient for you, accommodating your schedule.

Some Training Topics Include
- Auditing
- Basic Quality
- Engineering
- Education
- Healthcare
- Government
- Food Safety
- ISO
- Leadership
- Lean
- Quality Management
- Reliability
- Six Sigma
- Social Responsibility

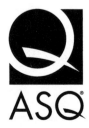

Visit www.asq.org/training for more information.